Working in Public Health

T0266293

Public health has always been central to the population's health and wellbeing, and people working in public health come from a wide range of disciplines and backgrounds. This practical and accessible book maps out comprehensively the range of exciting and varied options open to those considering a career in public health. Uniquely, it provides helpful information on how to become either a fully-fledged specialist or to work in an operational practitioner role.

This second edition provides an update on the variety of public health roles and the settings from which the workforce operates, with the inclusion of new material on climate change and sustainability. Written from a UK perspective, it nevertheless includes a chapter on working in international and global health. Each chapter is illustrated by career case studies and vignettes from people currently working in public health, illustrating their impact on improving or protecting the health of communities, as well as reducing inequalities.

In an era when the COVID-19 pandemic has thrown the spotlight on just how important public health roles are, this book should be essential reading for anyone aspiring to put public health at the heart of their own working life.

Fiona Sim trained in both general practice and public health and has held senior roles in public health, NHS management, education and the civil service. She has had a longstanding focus on building capacity and capability to improve health and reduce inequalities, including leading the establishment of voluntary regulation of public health specialists while at the English Department of Health. She is a former Chair of the Royal Society for Public Health, and was joint Editor-in-Chief of *Public Health* for 20 years until 2020. She was awarded an OBE for services to public health in 2015.

Jenny Wright's career spanned social work, research, NHS planning and management before she entered public health. She qualified as a specialist in public health in the early 2000s as soon as this was made possible for those from backgrounds other than medicine and ran a highly successful public health consultancy within the NHS. The latter part of her career was devoted to public health workforce development, focusing on developing the first UK-wide competence framework applicable to the whole public health workforce. She also led the work to develop and run the first UK public health careers website.

Working in Public Health
Choosing the Right Career
Second Edition

Edited by Fiona Sim and Jenny Wright

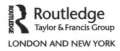
Routledge
Taylor & Francis Group

LONDON AND NEW YORK

Designed cover image: © Getty Images

Second edition published 2024
by Routledge
4 Park Square, Milton Park, Abingdon, Oxon, OX14 4RN

and by Routledge
605 Third Avenue, New York, NY 10158

Routledge is an imprint of the Taylor & Francis Group, an informa business

First edition published by Routledge 2015

British Library Cataloguing-in-Publication Data
A catalogue record for this book is available from the British Library

Library of Congress Cataloging-in-Publication Data
Names: Sim, Fiona, editor. | Wright, Jenny, 1948- editor.
Title: Working in public health : choosing the right career / [edited by] Fiona Sim and Jenny Wright.
Description: Second edition. | Milton Park, Abingdon, Oxon ; New York, NY : Routledge, 2024. | Includes bibliographical references and index.
Identifiers: LCCN 2023018924 (print) | LCCN 2023018925 (ebook) | ISBN 9781032560687 (hardback) | ISBN 9781032169743 (paperback) | ISBN 9781003433699 (ebook)
Subjects: LCSH: Public health--Vocational guidance--Great Britain.
Classification: LCC RA440.9 .W67 2024 (print) | LCC RA440.9 (ebook) | DDC 362.102341--dc23/eng/20230710
LC record available at https://lccn.loc.gov/2023018924
LC ebook record available at https://lccn.loc.gov/2023018925

ISBN: 978-1-032-56068-7 (hbk)
ISBN: 978-1-032-16974-3 (pbk)
ISBN: 978-1-003-43369-9 (ebk)

DOI: 10.4324/9781003433699

Typeset in Sabon
by KnowledgeWorks Global Ltd.

Contents

Foreword

Working to protect and improve the health of the public, whether in the UK or internationally, is one of the most socially useful, varied and intellectually interesting careers it is possible to have. People come into it from multiple routes, including medicine, academia, allied health professions and an increasing variety of career paths that demonstrate the diversity of roles relevant to public health. This book by distinguished practitioners and academics in public health allows people who are interested in a career in public health to explore the multiple options that are available, and the multiple career paths once they have made an initial decision to enter public health.

This book has been written in the shadow of the worst pandemic for at least a generation in COVID-19. It provided a vivid illustration of the importance of health protection, which aims to minimise the impact of infectious disease and other emergencies on the health of the population. It also, however, demonstrated the interconnectedness of public health, including health improvement and international health. Those who were most affected in the UK lived in the most deprived communities and had the highest burden of non-communicable diseases and risk factors such as obesity. The impact of measures to protect the population from COVID-19 had their greatest effect in the same populations living in deprived areas. The inequalities in health provision internationally and vulnerability to public health shocks of marginalised communities and poorer nations was put on vivid display. The power of science, and specifically public health science, and the contribution of academic analysis was also clearly demonstrated.

Between emergencies such as COVID-19 or HIV, public health continues to have remarkable impacts on society for the better. Often this requires the combination of technical skills and ability to operate across multiple levels in government. From the drive to improve sanitation in the 19th century through to the fight against the cigarette industry and its cynical attempt to addict children to a product which would kill them, and onto complex actions to reduce rising obesity, public health always needs to marry strong evidence with a determination to improve health compared to previous generations.

Those going into public health as a career need to have a realistic view of the difficulties they may face, and the changing nature of public health over time. While the numbers of nurses, surgeons or physiotherapists are largely predictable, public health is much more subject to changes in perceived need and current political settlement in national and local government. The size of the public health profession expands and contracts more than other areas of health. Entering public health therefore requires an ability to adapt and adjust to prevailing realities. The need, however, is constant for people with the skills to improve the health of the public at a population level, and an ability to seize opportunities to improve health as they arise.

Whether working in national government, local government, academia, the NHS, internationally or the wider health system, public health is a great career. It is possible to move between different parts of the system far more easily than many other areas of health, allowing for intellectual and practical variety. If you are thinking of moving into public health, this book allows you to see some of the breadth, excitement and impact on improving the health of society that can follow.

Christopher Whitty, Chief Medical Officer for England

Part 1
Introduction

1 Introduction to the book and to public health

Fiona Sim and Jenny Wright

Context

This book is an introduction to the infinitely varied world of public health careers. It will give you an understanding of what public health is, what issues the public health workforce needs to tackle and why they need tackling, and a description of some of the roles and career paths that public health professionals follow. Public health people are to be found in all walks of life, working in the public, independent and voluntary sectors. Many will make their contribution in overseas work with developing countries. We know you will be inspired to make your contribution even if you do not decide formally to enter public health! To get started, the book concludes with information and resources which are readily accessible and there to help.

The book is aimed at those who are starting on their career journeys in the UK and considering public health as an option, as well as those thinking about a move to public health in mid-career. It will also be of relevance and interest to those teaching on public health courses or providing careers advice as they prepare the next generation of public health practitioners and specialists. It is principally for people with a UK base. While it is the case that many of the core competencies required by the public health workforce will be similar across the world, the organisation of services and jobs available may be very different from one country to another. It is also the case that public health services find themselves subject to change quite frequently, so while we are confident the descriptions in this book are reasonably up to date in 2023, there will almost certainly be more change around the corner.

There are many definitions of 'public health'. The one most frequently used here dates from Sir Donald Acheson in 1988 and describes public health as 'the science and art of preventing disease, prolonging life and promoting health through the organised efforts of society', to which Derek Wanless added in 2004: 'through the organised efforts and informed choices of society, organisations, public and private, communities and individuals'.[1, 2] With these definitions, public health can be seen as the rightful consideration of the whole population. You can see that public health is very broad, and embraces the hugely diverse panoply of socioeconomic, educational, political

DOI: 10.4324/9781003433699-2

and healthcare or social care interventions that improve or protect the health and wellbeing of populations and communities.

Although we don't talk about it that much, the public health workforce is dedicated to making the world a better place, improving the health and wellbeing of the population and reducing inequalities. It does this through its understanding of the causes and impacts of disease and ill health on different communities. It achieves change, however, by working in partnership with other stakeholders. The social, environmental and economic factors determining health are complex and inter-related, and must always be taken into consideration in planning public health interventions. There are many different presentations of these factors. Figure 1.1 shows one well-known interpretation.

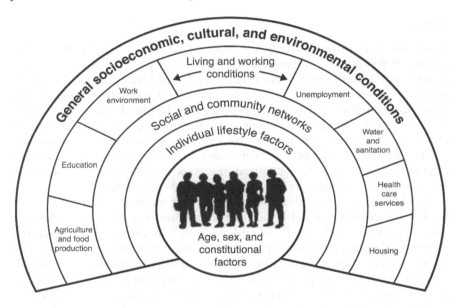

Figure 1.1 Dahlgren and Whitehead's Model of the Main Determinants of Health, 1991[3]

Reproduced with permission from the Institute for Futures Studies

Working in public health means aiming to make a real difference to people's lives. This is done in many different ways and in very varied settings. You will see that, unlike some other occupations, there is no single job that sums up 'the public health practitioner' or 'the public health specialist'. Public health professionals are to be found working throughout the system.

At local level:

- with individuals and families;
- with and for communities;

- with organisations that deliver services to individuals, families and communities, e.g.:

  - health services, including hospitals, primary care, community services, health boards, commissioners;
  - local authorities (local government);
  - social care;
  - education;
  - charities; and
  - independent/commercial sector organisations;

- in teaching and research (universities, colleges of higher education).

At regional and national levels:

- with organisations that plan and commission services and develop or shape policies, e.g.:

  - government departments and 'arm's length bodies';
  - regional or system level leadership of health services;
  - social care organisations;
  - charitable or community/3rd sector organisations;
  - some large independent/commercial companies;

At international and global levels:

- with organisations whose main focus is often improving health outcomes in low- or middle-income countries (e.g. charities, United Nations organisations, including the World Health Organization).

The rest of this introductory chapter outlines some of the major public health issues to be tackled, how we describe and define the public health workforce, a broad outline of careers in public health, what we mean by public health competence and the organisational structures within which the public health workforce operates across the UK in 2023. We conclude with an outline of the structure of the rest of the book.

A modern approach to evolving public health issues

What have public health professionals achieved for the population's health? In the UK, the public health movement really began in the middle of the nineteenth century in the face of outbreaks of what were then killer diseases, such as cholera and TB, and at a time of high infant mortality. The average life expectancy in England in the mid-nineteenth century was about 40 years, with around a quarter of children dying before they reached five years of age. The focus of nineteenth- and early-twentieth-century public health was, therefore, on understanding the causes of ill-health and enabling major legislation to achieve:

- clean water and sanitation;
- safe food;
- safe working conditions; and
- fewer outbreaks of infectious diseases.

In 1942, the main determinants of poor health were identified in the Beveridge Report as the 'Five Giants: Squalor, Ignorance, Want, Idleness, Disease'.[4] During the twentieth century, as the concepts of infection and contagious diseases became better understood, the central importance of clean water and sophisticated measures, such as immunisation programmes protecting whole populations, were also introduced.

Major public health achievements in the UK in the second half of the twentieth century were the Clean Air Act of 1956 and the introduction of seat-belt legislation in 1983 to promote safety on roads. In the twenty-first century, national measures to reduce the percentage of the population who smoke regularly, or prevent the harm caused to others by smokers, have been critical. In the 1960s, across the UK 70 per cent of men and 40 per cent of women smoked. Deaths caused by smoking were still in 2012 the largest avoidable cause of premature death and disability in the UK.[5] By 2019, the Office for National Statistics (ONS) reported that 14.1 per cent of the UK adult population were regular smokers.[6] There is still a considerable way to go and important threats to the health of the population, including (but this list is not exhaustive) from tobacco, alcohol, obesity, pandemics and poor air quality, continue to emerge or reappear.

Largely as a result of public health interventions, people are generally living longer than a century ago, but inequalities are marked within and between communities, and in some, little or no progress has been made. Living longer but in poor health is not most people's aspiration and remains a major challenge. There are far fewer infant and child deaths. In England, we speak of the north/south divide. Between 2018 and 2020, for example, life expectancy at birth for males was eight years less and for females seven years less in parts of north-west and north-east England compared with the wealthiest London boroughs.[7] Within London, similar differences in life expectancy are seen between the most affluent and poorest boroughs. And the COVID-19 pandemic has only exacerbated steadily worsening inequalities in health. The Marmot Review of December 2020 reported that not only did England have a higher rate of excess mortality than most of the rest of Europe, but it also took the most damaging economic hit.[8] This affected certain groups in society disproportionately.

So, in the early 2020s, there remain many tough challenges facing populations – and therefore the public health workforce and policy makers – and affecting all high-income countries, including the UK, and many middle- and lower-income countries, which include:

- continuing risks from new and emerging infectious diseases;
- management of non-communicable long-term conditions and the impact on healthcare needs of an expanding ageing population;
- climate change and its impact on health;
- rapidly evolving modern threats to public health, including obesity, lack of physical activity, poor nutrition and environmental air quality, as well as ongoing threats from tobacco and alcohol and other substance misuse;
- negative impacts specifically on mental health of adults and children; and
- huge inequalities in health status, as well as in access to healthcare, between and within populations.

Outside of pandemics (and, at the time of writing, the pandemic continues and we do not know the likely global death toll from COVID-19), deaths due to heart disease, stroke and cancer are the modern scourges. These are linked to societal changes which have led to worsening diets, increased access to alcohol and tobacco and lack of physical activity. Unfortunately, the dream of the founding fathers of the NHS, who thought that the population would steadily become healthier and the need for healthcare would diminish after 1948, was flawed as many people now live longer, but in poorer health. Those suffering from long-term conditions such as diabetes, circulatory diseases and dementia have a major impact on demand for health and social care. For the UK's public health workforce, one of the greatest current challenges, therefore, is to achieve more equitable healthy longevity – 'adding life to years as well as years to life'.[9]

As yet we do not know whether there will be a measurable impact on health in the UK as a result of leaving the European Union or what that might be, but we do know that collaborative research into health issues with EU partners is getting more difficult.

There is also uncertainty about the impact of the UK leaving the EU on how the COVID-19 pandemic has been handled. Pandemics do not respect national or any other borders, and the need for international collaboration has perhaps never been greater. Fortunately, research communities have been active internationally throughout the pandemic, including and beyond the EU. The UK's public health academics have been at the forefront of much pandemic-related research and development, but no single jurisdiction should view itself as self-sufficient and international collaborations have played an essential role in tackling the pandemic.

The pandemic experience has emphasised that the public health workforce must be prepared to meet all new challenges as and when they arise. For this, we need sufficient competent public health professionals with a voice at all levels and in all settings.

Specifically, the public health workforce will need:

- an awareness of differing health needs and how to identify and quantify them;
- knowledge of what influences our health and wellbeing;
- an understanding of how to prevent ill health and promote and protect health;
- an appreciation of ethics and the law and of political decision making;

And skills in:

- communicating risk effectively, including via the media;
- working successfully in collaboration with others to influence and negotiate with an awareness, since the pandemic, that communication may not necessarily be face-to-face;
- analysing and interpreting information on people and health; and
- reviewing literature to ascertain what interventions work and what will make a difference.

Above all, they will need to be able to work flexibly and quickly in response to changing issues and challenges. A focus on improving and tackling inequalities in the population's experience of health and wellbeing is at the heart of all public health practice.

Introducing the public health workforce

Public health is a multidisciplinary endeavour. Public health professionals come from a wide range of initial disciplines and backgrounds, which includes medicine, nursing and midwifery, other health disciplines such as pharmacy, nutrition, and other professions such as teaching, social work, or management. Increasingly, recruits to the public health workforce are from recent college and university graduates reflecting a wide range of science, humanities and arts subjects. The workforce embraces those just entering at the very start of their careers to senior strategic leaders and eminent professors.

Spheres of public health practice[10]

Public health practitioners and specialists usually work in one or more of several broad areas of practice. Understanding these will help to explain how a career in public health may be developed. Many people will end up working across two, three or more areas at some points during their careers.

The main areas of public health practice are as follows:

Improving health

Health improvement professionals work to improve people's health and wellbeing and prevent disease and ill health. This can involve working with individuals giving advice about healthy changes to their lifestyle, such as healthy eating or regular exercise, or with communities or the media to promote health campaigns such as regular teeth brushing or safer sex, commissioning and/or running health improvement programmes such as weight management or smoking cessation, or advocating for, and planning changes to, public health policy.

Examples of jobs in health improvement include smoking cessation advisers, community development officers, health promotion specialists, public health nurses, health visitors, public health pharmacists and health nutritionists.

Those considering health improvement careers may have enjoyed learning about education, human behaviour, sociology, psychology, marketing, communications, nursing or anthropology.

Protecting health

Health protection specialists and practitioners assure the safety of the population. This can involve protecting people from infectious diseases, including during epidemics and pandemics, but also in normal times, by mapping the course of an outbreak, tracing the origins, organising treatment and ongoing support, and communicating to the public about risks and safety measures. It can also include protecting people from environmental hazards, such as chemicals, radiation and noise, ensuring the safety of food or promoting safety within the workplace, such as fire safety or the safe handling of goods.

Examples of jobs in health protection include people employed as environmental health officers, infection control nurses, consultants in communicable disease control, laboratory staff and emergency planning staff.

Those considering health protection careers may have enjoyed particularly learning about biology, chemistry, epidemiology, environmental health, infectious diseases, laboratory techniques or engineering, but also other subjects such as geography and risk communication.

Maintaining and raising standards of health and social care

Healthcare public health professionals aim to raise the standards of services provided to the public to improve health outcomes and ensure services are safe, effective and efficient. Their work links closely to clinical care and might include developing specifications and setting priorities for others to provide primary preventive, screening or healthcare services across health and social care, evaluating and advising on quality and safety, as well as commissioning services, conducting research and providing evidence-based advice about what is likely to work best for the population in that locality.

Examples of healthcare public health jobs include quality or clinical governance or population health managers or technical officers, commissioning managers, research assistants and clinical effectiveness staff. At senior level, NHS Trust Medical and Nursing Directors often have executive responsibilities for many of these functions within their organisation, but these may not be identified explicitly as public health duties.

Those considering healthcare public health careers may have enjoyed especially learning about economics, research, business management, public policy, project management, clinical governance, and service evaluation and quality.

Working with information (health intelligence)

Health intelligence professionals collect, analyse, interpret and communicate information about health. This can relate to the general health and wellbeing of the whole population or it may consider the health status and needs of a particular section of the population, such as very elderly people. Accurate health intelligence analysis, as well as effective reporting and communication of the results to a variety of audiences, were essential public health tools during the pandemic. Just as important as the technical skills to retrieve and utilise data accurately is an understanding of data security, so that confidential or sensitive information about individuals is never incorrectly disclosed.

Examples of jobs include information analysts, epidemiologists, cancer intelligence officers and statisticians in health systems at every level.

Those considering health intelligence careers are likely to have enjoyed learning about mathematics, statistics, epidemiology, demography, ICT, basic sciences or database management.

Working in academic public health (teaching and research)

Academic public health involves investigating and teaching about public health issues. This can involve setting up, or working on, research projects to investigate one or more of a very broad range of issues, such as obesity, poor mental health, epidemics or climate change, and then publishing the findings so that others can learn in order to inform their own research or to influence some aspect of public policy. Many public health academics also teach about public health in their university.

Examples of jobs include professors of public health or epidemiology, lecturers, research fellows, research assistants and statisticians.

Those considering an academic public health career may have enjoyed particularly learning about research methods, epidemiology, demography, sociology, evidence-based policy and practice, humanities, evaluation and teaching.

Leading strategic planning, management and policy

People working in strategic roles provide leadership to public health work at different levels and for different organisations, national through to local, to improve the health and wellbeing of the population. They develop plans and the strategies to put those plans into action, then oversee implementation and evaluation, in order to understand their impact on whatever public health issue it was that they had set out to influence. Strategic leadership roles require tenacity, determination and perseverance, as well as an ability to be flexible, in order to see your objectives through to completion.

Examples of strategic leadership jobs include consultants, directors of public health and chief executive officers in any statutory, voluntary or independent sector organisation, where population health is an important goal.

Those considering careers in strategic management and leadership may have enjoyed learning about public policy, health services management, health scrutiny and how to communicate effectively. They will have gained experience of leadership and change management, as well as developing personal resilience, on their journey towards a strategic leadership position.

How we descrbe the public health workforce

There is no rigid definition of who is in the public health workforce. Often, the words 'public health' do not feature in job titles. The following three categories were developed in 2001 and probably still best describe the composition of the public health workforce.[11]

The wider workforce

This group includes those who have a role in health improvement, protecting health or reducing inequalities, but who would not necessarily regard themselves as part of the public health/health and wellbeing workforce.

This is the largest group in the workforce and includes front-line health professionals, social care and local government staff, including care assistants, teachers, nurses and social workers, who, through their interactions with patients or members of the public, provide advice on lifestyle or signpost people to further information, as well as elected members (e.g. councillors or members of parliament) and others, who through their political portfolios have influence over decisions that impact on people's health, such as planning or licensing regulations, provision of street lighting or leisure facilities.

Practitioners

Practitioners spend a major part or all of their time in operational public health practice. They usually work as part of multi-professional teams and include people who work with groups and communities, as well as individuals. They have knowledge and in-depth skills for their particular area of practice or public health domain.

This is the second largest group and includes the workforce responsible for much of the delivery of public health programmes, such as health promotion, public health nursing, public health nutrition and public health pharmacy, information on population health and demography and environmental health.

Some groups within this category will have formal professional qualifications, such as environmental health, nursing, pharmacy and nutrition. Others may be regulated through the UK Public Health Register (UKPHR) as practitioners. Many may have no formal public health qualification or registration.

Specialists

People in this group work at strategic or senior management level as consultants or specialists. Many have a high level of relevant technical expertise. At this level, ability to manage change, lead public health programmes and work across organisational boundaries are crucial, in addition to public health specialist technical skills.

This is the smallest group in the public health workforce. People working at this level are usually qualified in public health at specialist level and registered with one of the UK's three specialist public health regulatory bodies. For the purposes of this book, the emphasis will be on specialists and practitioners, the groups working at operational or strategic public health levels. It is important to remember, however, that people are often drawn in mid-career to a career in public health, having come (often without realising!) from what we have described here as the wider public health workforce.

Broad outline of careers in public health

Careers in public health are rewarding, challenging and also hugely varied. Entry routes can be confusing, however. The diagram in Figure 1.2 presents a simplified picture of the various ways in, and paths through, that someone aspiring to public health careers might choose to follow. For some practitioners, qualification routes are straightforward, such as those working in environmental health where there are specific courses, qualifications and regulation by the Chartered Institute of Environmental Health (CIEH) for England, Wales and Northern Ireland and by the Royal Environmental Health Institute of Scotland (REHIS). Public health nurses, who will include health visitors and school nurses, have all completed training as nurses or midwives and are regulated by the Nursing and Midwifery Council (NMC). Pharmacists, including public health pharmacists, are regulated through the General Pharmaceutical Council (GPhC). Those working as public health nutritionists can register with the UK Voluntary Register of Nutritionists (UKVRN).

For people completing their first degree, entry points are likely to be in administrative/assistant roles, from which valuable experience can be gained. More formal entry points can include health informatics apprenticeships run by the NHS for those leaving school and a more senior health and care intelligence specialist with entry following first relevant degree run by the Institute for Apprenticeships and Technical Education.[12] Health Education England (HEE) has also introduced Population Health Fellowships for NHS clinical staff in England.[13]

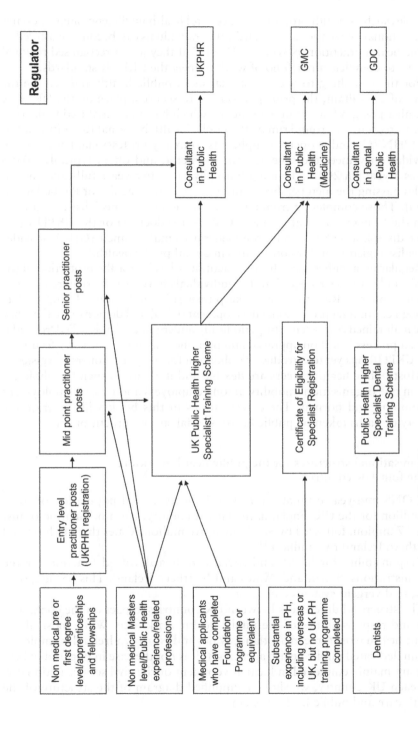

Figure 1.2 Formal routes to careers in public health

Roles such as health promotion officer and health intelligence analyst do not have national occupational standards, but individuals can become registered as public health practitioners with the UKPHR if they join a recognised regional scheme to complete a portfolio of work to meet the UKPHR standards.

For those wishing to become specialists in public health and achieve the status of consultant, the principal route is to secure a place on the UK-wide specialist postgraduate training scheme, which has an annual national, competitive recruitment round run by the Public Health National Recruitment Office (PHNRO) and is open to applicants from any professional background, provided they meet the scheme's entry criteria, and offers typically 60–90 places a year (in 2023). Training normally takes five years full-time and includes passing the membership examinations of the Faculty of Public Health (FPH). Those completing training are then eligible for specialist registration with the General Medical Council (GMC – for doctors) or the UKPHR (for other disciplines).[i] Separately, the General Dental Council (GDC) provides specialist registration for consultants in dental public health.[14]

Regulation at either specialist or practitioner level is for the protection of the public and provides recognition that individuals have met the required professional standards. Registrants must keep their skills and knowledge up to date through continuing professional development (CPD) and demonstrate that they have maintained competence by periodically undergoing what is called 'revalidation', a process based on appraisal and peer and patient/constituency feedback. The UKPHR has yet to introduce revalidation for the practitioners it registers.[ii]

Most public health careers are flexible and it is rare to spend a whole career in one organisation: mobility among employers and type of employment is common and normal. The career stories in this book will illustrate the variety of paths taken by public health specialists and practitioners.

Organisational structures for the public health workforce in the four UK countries

The ONS mid-year estimates for 2020 indicate a total population of some 67 million for the UK. England, the largest country, has a population of just over 57 million, followed by Scotland at five million, Wales three million and Northern Ireland two million.[15]

Responsibility for health and social care is a devolved function for the administrations in Scotland, Wales and Northern Ireland. This has led, over time, to divergent systems emerging.

The structural differences between UK countries impact on the configuration and responsibilities of the public health workforce. While most of the public health workforce in Scotland, Wales and Northern Ireland is employed within dedicated public health agencies, this is not the case in England, where staff are mainly employed in local government or the civil service nationally. For each UK country, we show a simplified diagram of the structure of the health care and public health systems.

England

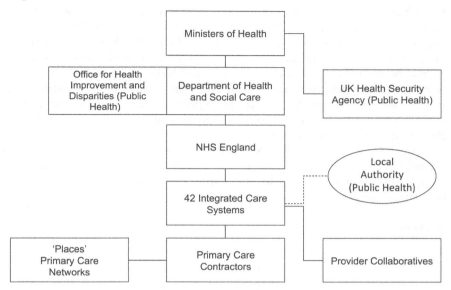

Figure 1.3 England

Recent NHS structural changes, effective from 2022, indicate a move away from competition towards collaboration and to develop, over time, a more integrated approach to planning and delivering health and social care and tackling inequalities. Since April 2022, 42 Integrated Care Systems (ICSs) in England, each covering a population of one to three million people, serve as the intermediate tier between the Department of Health and Social Care (DHSC) and local service providers (see Figure 1.3). ICSs have been statutory bodies since July 2022 as a result of the Health and Care Act 2022.

The goal is for ICSs to remove barriers between organisations to deliver better, more joined-up care for local communities. They bring together NHS providers, commissioners and local authorities to plan and organise collaboratively how health and care services are delivered in their area, taking over the commissioning function from the (former) Clinical Commissioning Groups (CCGs). Each ICS comprises partnerships of local organisations, including, for example, Primary Care Networks of GP practices, each network typically covering a population of 30,000–50,000 people. Community, mental health and acute hospital services are expected to group together to form provider collaboratives. The stated aim is to focus on improving population health outcomes, including prevention of diseases and addressing avoidable inequalities, by designing and delivering all health and care services for the local community within their financial allocation.[16] There is, however, no statutory public health board level position in ICSs.

Since the 2013 NHS reorganisation in England, the public health workforce has largely been split between local government or civil service employment (just a few public health staff are located within the NHS). Within upper-tier local authorities, a Director of Public Health heads up a team to provide health improvement programmes and public health advice and expertise both to the local authority and local NHS services, including supporting health protection. Each local authority with a public health team receives an annual grant for services to be provided, including sexual health, obesity, smoking cessation, physical activity and substance misuse. However, this grant may be used creatively.

Since 1 October 2021, the UK Health Security Agency (UKHSA) has led the health protection function nationally and the Office for Health Improvement and Disparities (OHID) located within DHSC leads national initiatives in England for population health improvement.

Scotland

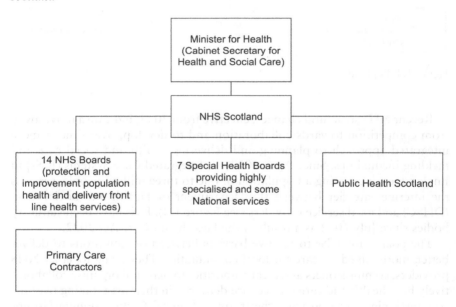

Figure 1.4 Scotland

The Scottish Government Department for Health and Wellbeing is responsible for NHS Scotland and for formulating and implementing health and community care policy (see Figure 1.4). NHS Scotland comprises 14 territorial NHS Boards, responsible for protection and improvement of their population's health and for the delivery of frontline health care services, seven Special NHS Boards covering all Scotland services such as ambulance, NHS Education and one public health body. This latter, Public Health Scotland, was launched on 1 April 2020 as the lead national agency for improving and protecting health and wellbeing. It has four key directorates for data-driven innovation, protecting health, place and wellbeing, and strategy, governance and performance.

Wales

Public Health Wales is one of a number of organisations that make up NHS Wales, formally established in 2009 (see Figure 1.5). Seven local health boards (LHBs) have a statutory responsibility for the health of their populations, planning, securing and delivering health care services. In addition, there are three NHS Trusts which deliver all-Wales services, comprising ambulance, cancer care and public health. There are in addition two Special Health Authorities which cover all of Wales – Digital Health and Care Wales and Health Education and Improvement Wales, plus support from the NHS Wales Shared Services Partnership. Each organisation is responsible to the Minister for Health and Social Services of the Welsh Assembly Government.

Public Health Wales employs 1,600 staff and is responsible for protecting and improving health and wellbeing and reducing inequalities for the people of Wales. It operates through seven directorates delivering all-Wales services, such as health protection, health and wellbeing, as well as local support. An Executive Director of Public Health is a formal member of each LHB supported by a team of public health staff. Memoranda of Understanding enable public health staff to work in partnership with other organisations.

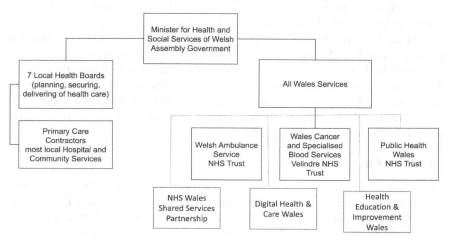

Figure 1.5 Wales

Northern Ireland

The Public Health Agency of Northern Ireland was established in 2009 as an executive agency of the Department of Health (see Figure 1.6). It is the lead national agency for improving and protecting health and wellbeing. It also provides public health support to commissioning and policy development, and health and social care research and development.

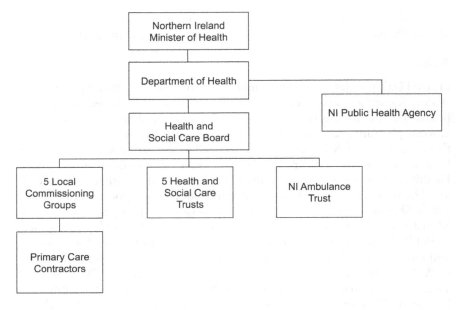

Figure 1.6 Northern Ireland

The Health and Social Care Board under the Department of Health is responsible for overall commissioning and managing services and resources. Five Local Commissioning Groups (LCGs) are responsible, on its behalf, for assessing health and social care needs, forming plans and securing the delivery from the five health and social care trusts whose boundaries they share. A sixth trust provides ambulance services across the country. Uniquely in the UK, health and social services are integrated in Northern Ireland. Each LCG has representatives from the Public Health Agency on it, as well as representatives from local government.

Structure of this book

Our aim is to share with readers a combination of practical information and personal narrative from our contributors, to help you to get a rich appreciation of the world of public health and about working in that world. One book cannot, on its own, cover all the possible roles and career options in public health. Rather, what the contributors have been enabled to do is to use their expertise as well as personal accounts to inspire and illustrate the opportunities. Their passion for their subject shines through, but they are honest accounts, not simply promotional material.

The book is divided into sections on different public health **functions** carried out by the public health workforce and the different **settings** from which they might operate. Each section commences with an introduction of what the future might hold in terms of challenges and opportunities, then describes working in that function or setting and the types of roles and skills needed, and concludes with one or more personal career stories from people with real life experience in the field. Contributions have come from all over Great Britain. All views expressed are the contributors' own. Many contributors have provided signposts to resources for interested readers to explore further. And, at the end of the book, we have included many more suggestions for additional reading and exploration. The final section covers entry to and options for training and development in public health careers.

Acknowledgements

We are grateful to Phil Mackie (Scotland) and Andrew Jones (Wales) for their help with their respective country organisational structures in this chapter and to Aminah Forknall for creating the images for country and careers diagrams. This book overall has only been made possible by the enthusiastic willingness of all the contributors to share their insights, expertise, experience, knowledge, passion and career stories. Many were written in the midst of the pandemic and we are particularly grateful for the trouble and care contributors took at this difficult time. We are indebted to all our contributors and delighted to bring this Second Edition to a wide readership, some of whom we are confident will be inspired as a result to work towards establishing their own successful public health careers. We are also grateful to the many other people who have encouraged us and shared their ideas freely, as well as suggesting contributors. We thank you all.

Notes

i For more information, see Part 4.
ii See Part 4 for more details.

References

1. Acheson, D. *Public Health in England: Report of the Committee of Inquiry into the Future Development of the Public Health Function*, Cm 289, London, HMSO, 1988.
2. Wanless, D. *Securing Good Health for the Whole Population, Final Report*, London, HMSO, 25 February 2004.
3. Dahlgren, G. and Whitehead, M. *Policies and Strategies to Promote Social Equity in Health*, Stockholm, Institute for Futures Studies, 1991.
4. Beveridge, W. (Chair). *Social Insurance and Allied Services* (SIAS), Cmd 6404, London, HMSO, 1942.
5. Royal College of Physicians and UK Centre for Tobacco Studies. *Fifty Years since Smoking and Health*, RCP, March 2012. Available at: www.rcplondon.ac.uk/projects/outputs/fifty-years-smoking-and-health.
6. ONS. *Adult Smoking Habits in the UK: 2019*, Statistical Bulletin, release date 7 July 2020.
7. Raleigh, V. *What Is Happening to Life Expectancy in England?* 6 December 2021. Available at: www.kingsfund.org.uk/publications/whats-happening-life-expectancy-england.

8. Marmot, M., Allen, J., Goldblatt, P., Herd, E. and Morrison, J. *Build Back Fairer: The COVID-19 Marmot Review*, The Health Foundation, December 2020. Available at: www.health.org.uk/publications/build-back-fairer-the-covid-19-marmot-review.

9. McKee, M. and Krentel, A. (eds). *Issues in Public Health: Challenges for the 21st Century*, 3rd edn, Maidenhead, Open University Press, 2022.

10. The Faculty of Public Health in its Good Public Health Practice Framework of 2016 cites three public health domains of Health Improvement, Health Protection and Healthcare Public Health. It includes three underlying functions: public health knowledge and intelligence; academic public health; and workforce development. Available at: www.fph.org.uk/media/1305/short-guide_good-public-health-practice_april-2016.pdf.

11. Donaldson, L. *Report of the Chief Medical Officer's Project to Strengthen the Public Health Function in England*, London, Department of Health, 2001.

12. NHS. *NHS Apprenticeships*. Available at: www.healthcareers.nhs.uk/career-planning/study-and-training/apprenticeships/nhs-apprenticeships; Institute of Apprentices & Technical Education. *Health and Care Intelligence Specialist*, 2021. Available at: www.instituteforapprenticeships.org/apprenticeship-standards/health-and-care-intelligence-specialist-v1-0.

13. Health Education England. *Population Health Fellowships Created to Support Integrated Care*, 21 January 2020. Available at: www.hee.nhs.uk/news-blogs-events/news/population-health-fellowships-created-support-integrated-care.

14. Note that dentists have a separate, but equivalent, specialist training scheme in dental public health and are regulated by the General Dental Council (GDC). The other, exceptional, routes to registration as a public health specialist are via retrospective portfolio assessment for those who have substantial experience in public health, but who, for a justifiable reason, have not completed specialist training in the UK. For doctors, this would be via the GMC's Certificate of Eligibility for Specialist Registration (CESR) route and, for non-medics, via the UKPHR.

15. ONS. *Population Estimates*, 25 June 2021. Available at: www.ons.gov.uk/peoplepopulationandcommunity/populationandmigration/populationestimates#timeseries.

16. NHS Providers. *Integrated Care Systems Explained: Making Sense of the New NHS Structure*, 2022. Available at: https://nhsproviders.org/media/691164/system-working-glossary-for-governors.pdf.

Websites relating to UK public health structures

Office for Health Improvement & Disparities (OHID) leads the health improvement and inequalities function. Available at: www.gov.uk/government/organisations/office-for-health-improvement-and-disparities.

Public Health Agency, Northern Ireland, is responsible for public health improvement, health protection, health and social care commissioning, advice and research and development. Available at: www.publichealth.hscni.net.

Public Health Scotland is the lead national agency for improving and protecting health and wellbeing. Available at: www.publichealthscotland.scot.

Public Health Wales is the national public health service for Wales. Available at: https://phw.nhs.wales/.

UK Health Security Agency (UKSHA) leads the health protection function and deals with the threat of infection. Available at: www.gov.uk/government/organisations/uk-health-security-agency.

Part 2

Public health functions

Fiona Sim and Jenny Wright

Introduction

This section outlines the diversity of essential functions carried out by the public health workforce for challenges to population health and wellbeing to be met. For each function, there is an expert viewpoint on future challenges and opportunities, followed by an overview of the function, what it actually does and how to gain experience in it, bearing in mind that public health professionals might work in a variety of settings. Each function concludes with accounts of personal career journeys to give the reader a picture of real-life experiences, wherever possible, from a specialist and from a practitioner in the field; but you will see that most people have worked in more than one of these functions during their career.

The public health functions included in this section are:

- health improvement and prevention;
- health intelligence;
- health and social care services;
- health protection;
- academic public health;
- international and global health; and
- climate change and sustainability.

DOI: 10.4324/9781003433699-3

2 Health improvement and promotion

Kevin Fenton; Dona Milne; Cathy Steer;
Ashley Gould; Yeyenta Osasu; Fiona Sim;
Jenny Wright

Introduction to this function

Health improvement professionals work actively to promote and improve people's health and wellbeing. This can involve working with individuals, communities, whole populations and policy makers. Often, the work has focused on 'downstream' behaviour and lifestyle interventions to bring about change. In recent decades, the emphasis has shifted to consideration of major 'upstream' social determinants of health, such as education, employment, housing and income, for which there is sound evidence of the positive impact of interventions at population level.

During the pandemic, particularly in 2020 and 2021, many health improvement programmes had to be placed 'on hold' as the public health workforce redirected its efforts to health protection. During this time, inequalities worsened with the deleterious effects of lockdowns and often economic hardship on both mental and physical health and wellbeing. The contributions that follow will include reflections about the impact of the pandemic on their work and what needs to happen next.

Future challenges and opportunities – a vision for public health improvement

Kevin Fenton, Regional Director London, Office for Health Improvement and Disparities (OHID)

COVID-19 has shone a light on longstanding and acutely exacerbated health, social and economic inequalities. As we enter the pandemic's third year, global vaccine and treatment equity, health systems strengthening and resilience, pandemic preparedness and response, sustainable economic recovery and climate justice will undoubtedly dominate our public health priorities. These priorities exist within the context of fundamental shifts in the public's understanding and engagement around health, social and political polarisation, declining trust in government and institutions, and growing influence of social media on our attitudes, behaviours, values and beliefs.

DOI: 10.4324/9781003433699-4

Taken together, these priorities and contexts require an evolution in our understanding and practice of public health. One that places public health specialists and practitioners and approaches at the centre of policy and programmatic responses, ensuring evidence-informed action, agile responsiveness, delivery at scale, leadership within complex adaptive systems and a resolute focus on tackling inequalities. Undoubtedly, the leadership lessons acquired throughout the pandemic provide strong foundations for this transformation and include a renewed commitment to: place-based leadership; stronger actions by anchor institutions (hospitals, universities, local government, etc.) in addressing social and structural determinants of ill health; robust community engagement; and investment in our public health workforce.

We have seen the critical importance of 'place' in defining the assets, resources, partnerships, leadership and advocacy required to improve health and tackle inequalities.[i] Public health specialists and practitioners must continue to play a lead role in creating and sustaining place-based leadership for health, through collaborative networks, governance, partnerships and ways of working, delivered at the appropriate level(s) of geographic or organisational aggregation. Place-based leadership is critical for establishing the vision, strategy, governance and accountability for improving health and tackling inequalities. This type of systems leadership is based on negotiation and influence rather than direction and is often best developed through teams rather than individuals, involving a guiding coalition taking responsibility to lead system-wide change.

Our anchor institutions (those organisations which have an important presence in a place, by being largescale employers or commissioners of local services) are a key component of place-based responses to improving health and have played a critical role throughout the pandemic, enabling those people involved in the delivery of essential services to take broader actions to improve the wellbeing of local communities. Future opportunities in place include strengthening the delivery of effective prevention interventions, employee health and wellbeing, community engagement and empowerment, workforce training and development, and sustainable economic development. Public health efforts to develop, clarify and strengthen the role of anchor institutions will be key to accelerating improvements in population health and keeping inequalities and prevention firmly on the agenda.

Communities really matter for health and evidence shows that communities that are vibrant, socially connected, engaged and empowered are healthier and more resilient. The COVID-19 pandemic has reinforced the reality that sustained improvements in health are unachievable without local communities being fully engaged, trusting and involved in co-creating solutions for the issues that matter to them. We must build on the strong community-centred models for improving health that have developed throughout the pandemic to help tackle other health challenges, supporting local people to have better control over their lives, develop good social connections and live in healthy, safe neighbourhoods. Public health's role in advocacy, funding and support for these asset-based community approaches for improving health will be critical.

No vision for the future of health improvement would be complete without a resolute focus on workforce training and development, ensuring public health specialists and practitioners have the skills, tools and confidence required for the challenges ahead. The nature, range and magnitude of the challenges ahead will require us to act differently to achieve different (and better) outcomes. Our technical competencies must be complemented by equal investment in leadership and management development to include more effective listening and engagement skills, leading across organisational boundaries, managing conflict, empowering others, working in political environments, evaluating proposed solutions, and leveraging data, information and insights for action. We need to establish where, and how, public health expertise can best be deployed to achieve the greatest heath impact and establish clear evidence-based and ethical priorities on maximising the use of scarce resources.

I have been privileged to work with and to lead public health research, policy development and programmes over the past three decades and I have seen first-hand the tremendous contributions of specialists and practitioners in addressing society's problems. In the wake of COVID-19, the challenges and opportunities that lie before us are unprecedented. Yet the pandemic also opens the possibility for our profession to be an integral part of recovery, with ambitious new agendas for the nation's health and wellbeing. We now need to create the right conditions for effective local action with public health at the centre, helping to clarify systems' ambitions, creating a shared understanding of the change desired, promoting more active, community-centred intervention, and supporting improvements with data and evaluation.

Overview of the health improvement function

*Dona Milne, Director of Public Health, NHS Lothian and Cathy Steer,
Head of Health Improvement, NHS Highland, Scotland*

What we mean by health improvement

The term 'health improvement', often called 'health promotion', is used to describe any type of activity that leads to an improvement in health outcomes for the population. Historically, health improvement was often limited to what we would call behaviour and lifestyle changes, such as increasing physical activity and eating a healthy diet. These issues were often perceived as individualistic and aimed at those who were able to make changes in their lives. Many of these programmes were successful at an individual level, but didn't always lead to changes at a population level, which is ultimately what public health teams are trying to achieve. These programmes continue, but now there is greater recognition that traditional health improvement programmes alone will not improve health and that a greater focus is needed on the wider determinants of health.

Recently, in Scotland, we have moved towards talking more about prevention and population health, where we have a wider understanding of the social determinants of health and how improvements in people's life circumstances lead to improvements in health. This can include those more traditional health improvement elements, but we also need an increased focus on education, employment, housing, reducing poverty and increasing income, which have significant impacts on longer-term health outcomes.

Population health function

Public health in Scotland is delivered by both specialist teams trained in public health and partners who work in broader areas of population health, such as those who work within Health and Social Care Partnerships, the NHS, local authorities and the third sector.[ii] In Scotland, public health teams are still based in the NHS, although some health improvement functions are within Health and Social Care Partnerships (NHS and Local Authority), unlike England, where public health teams were moved back to local authorities in 2012. Specialist public health teams are either part of a local NHS board, of which there are 14 in Scotland, or part of Public Health Scotland, the national public health agency.

Wherever a health improvement specialist works, they are likely to be part of a multi-disciplinary team that includes data and health intelligence specialists, nurses, consultants and administrators with specialist training and experience of working in public health.

Most of the work of public health teams is undertaken in partnership with others. Many of the levers for change do not sit with public health teams: they sit elsewhere, such as in local authorities or in communities themselves. There are structures within Scotland that can facilitate partnership working across systems to reduce inequalities and improve health. There is already integration of health and social care (https://hscscotland.scot/hscps/) and public health teams often work with those local services to consider how to ensure services are accessible, reaching those who are most disadvantaged and supporting the delivery of high-quality services.

There are also local Community Planning Partnerships[1] which bring together all public and third-sector agencies to agree a Local Outcome Improvement Plan (LOIP) for each local authority area in Scotland. There are 32 local authority areas in Scotland and the joint working across partners due to the creation of these Community Planning Partnerships can lead to significant changes in local places that improve outcomes for the population. This can include work on housing, transport, green spaces and employability programmes. Local public health partnerships can play a key role involving specialist public health teams, working as part of the wider public health workforce and linking across the system to influence improvements in population health.

What population health contributes to health outcomes

Not all ill health can be prevented by health services. Some of the biggest gains in health improvement are as a result of changes to the circumstances in which people are born, grow, work and live: think of historical changes like the provision of clean water, reduction in poor housing and access to universal education – these have all made significant differences to health outcomes. Improving life circumstances are some of the most important things that we can do to improve health, as it can prevent ill health from occurring in the first place.

It can be difficult to see where public health has made a difference in the short term: it can often take many years before the impact of changes are evident. We have identified two examples which we think show a clear difference that has been made by public health: teenage pregnancy and smoking.

- Numbers of teenage pregnancies in Scotland in the late 1990s were much higher than in similar countries in Western Europe. There was recognition that many young women were missing out on completing their education due to an early pregnancy, which was leading to a cycle of deprivation for them and their children. Health Improvement teams in Scotland worked with local and national partners to review the evidence of what could make a difference to these young women and how we could achieve a delay in very early pregnancies. A combination of relationships and sexual education, alongside access to high-quality sexual health services designed for young people, were identified as essential components of any intervention, and work was taken forward across Scotland to deliver these. However, the thing that many of us feel made an even bigger impact on the reduction we subsequently saw on teenage pregnancies was an increased focus on school attendance, educational attainment and local community activities. It may seem strange to say this, but the cause of teenage pregnancies isn't just unprotected sex – it is also poverty, and a more holistic approach was therefore required.
- Adult smoking prevalence in Scotland has fallen from 31% in 1999 to 28% in 2003 to 17% in 2019. There is extensive evidence that smoking is one of the leading preventable causes of ill health and early death. Public health has been at the forefront of taking effective action to help people to stop smoking, prevent people from starting to smoke and protect people from second-hand smoke. Like many public health issues, reducing the prevalence of smoking requires a range of population-wide strategies and success is not achieved through any one measure, but rather through a multi-faceted approach that balances a range of national and local action. Recognising that smoking rates remain disproportionately high in the

most deprived areas – 40% compared to 11% in the least deprived areas, comprehensive tobacco control programmes also need to recognise the importance of tackling the wider determinants of health, including poverty, income, employment, housing and education. A broad multi-pronged public health approach that has included support for people to stop smoking combined with a range of local and national actions to implement smoke-free policies in workplaces/public places, introduction of a ban on advertising and display of tobacco products, inclusion of tobacco control in the school curriculum, price rises on tobacco products and other actions have been instrumental in changing social attitudes to smoking and reducing the prevalence and therefore associated ill health from smoking. Figure 2.1 outlines the range and timing of a number of actions to reduce smoking and the changing prevalence of smoking in Scotland.

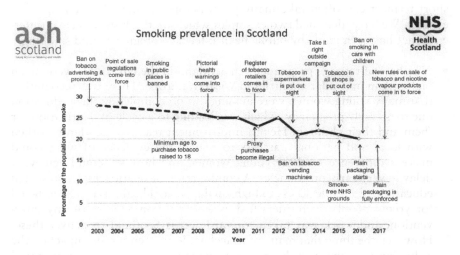

Figure 2.1 Actions to reduce the prevalence of smoking in Scotland

Diagram produced with permission from Ash Scotland and Public Health Scotland

Skills and qualifications needed to work in health improvement

The skills and qualifications required for a role in health improvement are wide ranging. They relate to the overall function of public health: to improve and protect the public's health and to reduce health inequalities between individuals, groups and communities through coordinated system-wide action. Use of data and intelligence is important to inform health improvement programmes, including measuring, monitoring and reporting population health and wellbeing, identifying health needs and risks to health, and describing inequalities in health and use of services. Everyone undertaking a role in health improvement will be involved in carrying out some work that is about sourcing and using data to inform development of interventions or to review or evaluate interventions or services.

To be effective, health improvement programmes and projects should be informed by evidence. Therefore, having the skills to access, evaluate and apply evidence to plan the delivery of health improvement interventions or services is important. Often health improvement practitioners are required to translate national or local policy and strategy into effective health improvement action. Supporting implementation of policy and strategy to improve health and wellbeing and reduce inequalities is an important skill in a health improvement role.

Partnership working is a crucial part of delivering health improvement programmes and having strong collaboration skills is essential to a role in health improvement. These skills are applied in many different settings, including collaborating directly with communities, working with partners across public sector organisations and joining forces with a wide range of services and service users.

Project management skills are important in planning and implementing health improvement interventions, from defining goals to setting timescales and milestones, to monitoring progress and evaluating interventions. Communication skills are at the core of a career in health improvement and are essential for informing, influencing and motivating individuals, communities and organisations.

There is no specific training course, vocational qualifications or set requirements to enter a career in health improvement, although there are relevant university courses that can help prepare you, including courses in health improvement/promotion, public health policy or health studies. A basic requirement is a degree in a health or related subject or equivalent experience. Other relevant subjects that can be helpful include psychology, behavioural science, nursing or midwifery, social sciences, education or community development. People taking up roles in health improvement come from a variety of backgrounds and have a range of qualifications in nursing, teaching, community education, physiotherapy, dietetics, social work and a variety of other related disciplines.

To progress to senior roles in health improvement, it is often necessary to gain a Master's level qualification in Health Improvement/Promotion, Public Health or a subject closely related to the practice of health improvement. Registration for non-medical public health professionals is currently voluntary, but increasingly employers are looking for registration with the UK Public Health Register, either through the practitioner or specialist registration schemes.[iii]

Gaining some relevant experience in a public health-related area can help you to move into a health improvement role. This could include working with communities or groups, or working in a data or intelligence role. Relevant work experience can be in health, education, social care, community development or a range of other disciplines and experience can be gained working in settings including the NHS, local authority and third- or community-sector organisations. However, if you want to move into a career in health improvement, you will need to demonstrate that you have an understanding of and have used health promotion principles, theories, models and approaches. At the end of 2022, there were no specific apprenticeship schemes for health improvement in Scotland. However, this is a route that is likely to develop in the near future.

The type of roles found in public health teams

Health improvement roles influence national policy and enable national policy to be put into practical local actions. In collaboration with a diverse range of stakeholders, both at local and national level, the focus and effort ultimately is to improve population health outcomes and to reduce inequalities.

There are a range of health improvement roles and career opportunities that require the generic skills outlined in the previous section. Generic health improvement roles are increasingly available in national organisations like Public Health Scotland and in local systems with opportunities mainly found in NHS Board Public Health Departments, Health and Social Care Partnerships and Local Authorities. Depending on the level of post, these roles generally focus on particular health issues like mental health or physical activity or on life stages like the early years or children and young people. They can also focus on settings like schools or health services or take a place-based approach. Whatever the portfolio, generic health improvement roles provide specialist health improvement strategic and operational leadership and support to colleagues and partners to deliver health improvement projects and programmes.

The role of communities in improving health is increasingly being recognised as a significant factor in national health policy. The priorities to improve public health in Scotland include a focus on community and place and a commitment to improving health through a joined-up approach with communities as an important element of 'whole system working'. Community health is a core component of the work of local health improvement teams and increasingly there is a need to focus health improvement efforts at a community level. Community health improvement practitioners use a series of approaches based on the principles of community development to support local communities to improve health through building social capital, strengthening resilience, utilising community assets and including communities in decision making.

Health Improvement Advisor roles support people to identify and address their holistic health and wellbeing needs. The role tends to be focused on delivery of individual or group-based health improvement interventions, including assessing, advising and supporting people to stop smoking or achieve a healthy weight through modifying lifestyle factors such as diet and physical activity. Health Information and Resources Officers are responsible for supporting health improvement initiatives and services by sourcing, recommending and providing accurate, up-to-date health information and resources to the public and professionals. This can include written materials, such as leaflets and posters, as well as activity materials, educational games, models and other resources for use by health and social care services, at health and community events and in schools. Increasingly, the role involves sourcing and providing online information and resources and supporting local health information social media sites. Health Information and Resources Officers are sometimes involved in providing and operating health information telephone helplines that support people to access health improvement interventions by signposting them to, for example, stop smoking, healthy weight and infant feeding services.

Why public health can be a rewarding career

For those of us who dislike unfairness and recognise that it isn't poor decision making by individuals and communities that lead to poor health but poor policies that lead to ill health, public health can be a very rewarding career. Many of us who join public health teams have come from frontline services where we feel that we are only addressing the symptoms and not the causes of poor health outcomes and we want to make a difference. Public health provides an opportunity to look further upstream at effective approaches that aim to prevent ill health in the first place.

Public health is in the limelight more than ever before due to the COVID-19 pandemic – the public perhaps understands who we are and what we do more than they ever did before. We have an opportunity to use that recognition and influence to shape public policy and future interventions towards a focus on improving life circumstances. We learned a lot about doing this at pace during the pandemic and it is essential that we bring that pace to addressing inequalities. We have a responsibility to do this and if this fits with what you would like to see happen, a career in public health could be a good choice.

Working in health improvement provides an opportunity to develop a wide range of skills and competencies. No two days are the same and one of the great attractions to a career in health improvement is the variety and opportunities available to work on different public health issues in a number of settings with a range of people and organisations. Often there is no typical working day, but most days may include meeting with partners or stakeholders, advocating for action to improve health, developing project or programme plans, writing briefings, developing strategies, policy or guidelines, researching evidence or best practice, reviewing data and information, or developing or delivering training. Working in health improvement is extremely rewarding as the role is about facilitating change and having a positive impact on the health of individuals and communities. It can sometimes be challenging to explain public health evidence (to policy makers as well as the public) and change can take time, but hang in there: amazing things can happen!

My career journey – Cathy Steer

My career started in Nutrition and Dietetics where I had the opportunity to work in hospital and community settings. I found myself drawn to working in communities and enjoyed the varied opportunities to work with them on a wide range of food and health projects. I moved into public health to take on a role as Heart Health Officer with a portfolio of work that covered healthy eating, physical activity and smoking. Although initially the focus of my work was on lifestyle issues, I was able to develop my knowledge and skills in public health and health improvement principles, theories and practice, which helped me gain more senior roles in public health and broaden my portfolio of work, including getting involved in work on health inequalities, community health development and health promoting in schools. After completing my Master's in Health Improvement and Promotion, I was able to secure a leadership role in public health as Head of Health Improvement. Taking on a public health leadership role has been one of the most rewarding roles of my career. I have been able to have strategic influence over a wide range of health improvement programmes, champion health inequalities within my own and partner organisations, influence and develop national and local public health strategy and policy, and build a team of health improvement specialists who deliver a wide range of health improvement programmes. I continue to enjoy the challenge of working in an area where there is constant change and development. Despite being in this role for a number of years, no two days are ever the same and I continue to develop my public health knowledge and skills, with every day being a 'school learning day'.

My career journey – Dona Milne

My career started in community education with a focus on youth work and community development. I worked initially within a local authority education department and then the third sector locally and nationally. All of my roles seemed to have a focus on health improvement and reducing inequalities and I realised that was an area I was interested in. I moved into the NHS to lead a large sexual health demonstration programme for the Scottish Government and through that became interested in public health. I was very fortunate to be able to retrain in public health while also working for the NHS. Over a number of years, I was able to participate in a portfolio of accreditation for senior public health staff and subsequently took on the role of Public Health Specialist, followed by an appointment as a Public Health Consultant. During that time, I worked in a local health board and Scottish Government. I took on the role of Deputy Director of Public Health alongside consultant duties, and then became a Director of Public Health in 2018. After 21 years in public health, I can thoroughly recommend it.

Career stories

Ashley Gould, Public Health Consultant, NHS Wales

'We're all a product of our environments.'

Getting started on my career in public health

It happened by accident in many respects – I didn't really know what I wanted to do when in 6th form college studying A-Level biology, chemistry and maths, and eventually followed the lead of a slightly older friend and got onto a BSc Honours course in Environmental Health. From day one, I knew I had made the correct career choice – the variety of the discipline, the opportunity to make a tangible difference to people's lives (I always wanted to 'save the world'!) and perhaps the vocational certainty really hooked me in. These aspects fuelled my interest and increased understanding around how we are all a product of our environments, and how personal characteristics, social connections and norms – and our living, learning, working and home spaces – contribute to our wellbeing, perhaps (and it's proven to be so at a population level: www.who.int/news-room/questions-and-answers/item/determinants-of-health) more than the healthcare services we call on from time to time. The degree course was a 'sandwich' – with periods outside university doing-the-doing in a local authority – helping to demonstrate the tangible difference that could be made to people's environments and their health. It was a degree that was vocational – but still had breadth – food safety, health and safety, pollution control (air, land and water) and improving housing to standards that were 'fit for human habitation'.

My first job was as an Environmental Health Officer (Public Health and Housing) in Luton Borough Council – 'public health' here reflected the long-lasting legacy of 'the first wave' of public health in the late 1800s![2] It meant resolving threats to health from water and sanitation – overflowing cesspits and septic tanks (they are different in law), public and private sewer faults (they are also different in law) and resolving 'statutory nuisances' – a selection of factors included in the then ground-breaking Environmental Protection Act 1990 that were 'prejudicial to health or a nuisance', and included smoke, smells or noise coming from premises and accumulations/deposits (of refuse, etc.). As well as knowing when to use enforcement powers (more than the police have), I learned the art of diplomacy and the need for analysis, and developed the attributes of persistence and optimism – to make a difference to people's life circumstances, and many of the determinants of health.

Early experience in public health, relevant courses and qualifications obtained

My most valuable early experience was dealing with people – what matters to them, and how to work with them – 'public servant' experience. This included interacting with civic leaders (councillors), complainants, tenants and landlords (of dangerous rented houses and of dangerous noisy pubs) – and using the range of tools, interventions and treatments at my disposal to improve living conditions and reduce risks to health – legislation, persuasion and education. After my initial BSc Honours Degree in Environmental Health (due in part to the efforts of my wife, who I met on the course and who coached me through), I pursued qualifications in environmental law, and obtained a Post Graduate Diploma in Acoustics and Noise Control.

Public health posts held

I moved to Environmental Health Officer posts in Berkshire and, in sharp contrast to that, Sandwell in the West Midlands, covering actions to improve housing conditions for (means-tested) owner-occupiers and those in privately rented accommodation – through enforcement activity and overseeing grant-funded improvement work. I had a portfolio of multi-occupied houses to 'look after', often occupied by those most disadvantaged in society. My role involving making properties safe to live in – investigating a fatal fire in such a property and taking the landlord to court underlined 'the why', and stuck with me (and motivated me) for years. I was also involved in the adaptation of homes for disabled residents, working with Occupational Therapists to sustain independence and in noise control – night-time nuisance enforcement, neighbourhood disputes about barking dogs, unceasing alarms in unoccupied buildings, and minimising the impact (on health, including sanity) of ground-shaking drop-forges and demolition activity.

I then moved into the policy arena – first as a Health Alliance Co-ordinator, working in the white-space between local authorities, health agencies and third-sector bodies – on health improvement (known as health promotion back then) and social care interfaces. Moving to a Policy Officer (Health Improvement) role in the Welsh Local Government Association (WLGA) at a time of increasing overlap with the National Public Health Service for Wales, particularly around the wider determinants of health and wellbeing, and working to squeeze the biggest collaborative advantage out of the system in terms of primary prevention of disease. I eventually led a national team in the WLGA, acting as a focal point for the development and delivery of local Health, Social Care and Wellbeing strategies – providing the interface between government and local partnerships, shaping guidance and sustaining networks of practice. I was inducted into the analytical, trusted, optimistic, persistent responsibilities of being a Consultant in Public Health at this point, through having a final year Specialty Public Health Registrar (StR), who was a GP by background, spending six months in my Health Improvement Team. She convinced me I could make a difference as a Consultant in Public Health, and encouraged me to apply for the public health training scheme.

My StR journey started with the bang of interviewing Executive Directors from each health board in Wales and a range of other people, as part of a Ministerial review of child safeguarding policy and practice. I co-authored a report with recommendations that were ultimately enshrined in guidance, and remain in place. A Master's Degree in Public Health gave me so much more of the 'know-how' around epidemiology, research methods, disease causation, gathering and using data and intelligence, social policy and health economics, and the organisation and management of health and health care – a range of disciplines wider than Environmental Health! The 'show-how' happened through projects, including: around screening for liver cancer and discussions with the NHS Liver Tsar; responding to Ebola risk in miners returning to the UK from West Africa; and ending up on TV encouraging Mumps Measles and Rubella (MMR) vaccine uptake while dealing with a measles outbreak. I piloted the mapping of alcohol sales outlet density and alcohol-related harm, championed smoking cessation for cardiac patients, acted as a Consultant in Public Health (at a critical year-end) and developed the 'MyBetterHealth' prescription, with GPs and a cardiologist – so they could 'prescribe' preventive actions. The range of opportunities and the time to learn was an absolute privilege.

My first substantive Consultant role was as national lead for tobacco control – transitioning 'Stop Smoking Wales' to 'Help Me Quit', developing and introducing minimum service standards, continuing service delivery throughout the pandemic (shifting all services to tele-med delivery) and applying behavioural science as part of a programme that secured a Europe-wide award for social marketing. More importantly than all of that was being part of a system that delivered five years' consecutive growth in the proportion of smokers in Wales choosing to try to quit with NHS support (the proven most effective route). During this period, I also gained an interest in quality improvement methodologies and became an Improvement Advisor after studying with the Institute for Healthcare Improvement based in Boston, USA.

From early March 2020, along with nearly everyone else working in public health, I switched to deploying my knowledge, skills and time almost entirely to tackling the SARS CoV-2 virus (the COVID-19 pandemic). I spoke with the self-isolating families of the first case in Wales; was involved with contact tracing the first 20 cases; establishing an Enclosed Settings Cell, working tirelessly to support care homes; and led a Behaviour Change Cell (producing system-wide guidance to help optimise communications). This work led to me co-chairing the Risk Communication and Behaviour Insights Sub Group of the Welsh Government's Technical Advisory Group – shaping the strategic 'Keep Wales Safe' approach, and wide-ranging policy and practice to optimise widespread adoption of personal protective behaviours, including through guidance: 'Sustaining COVID-safe behaviours in Wales' and 'Living safely with COVID-19 in Wales: risk communication and behavioural science perspectives'.

In all of these posts, I have strived to make a difference to life circumstances and prevent disease.

What I enjoy about my current role

I'm currently Programme Director of a new Behavioural Science Unit in Public Health Wales – developing a hub of specialist expertise on behavioural science, and developing the increased understanding of the psychological, cognitive, social and environmental determinants of behaviours/decisions – to shape the design of policy, services, and communications to improve health and wellbeing. The range, opportunity and impact of this work, around the climate crisis, communicable disease, health-harming behaviours and health screening (as a starter list!) is energising. I've co-authored a guide to using behavioural science and supported the World Health Organization's efforts in this arena, contributing to guidance on setting up Behavioural Insights (BI) units and further developing the field.[3]

Maintaining a work/life balance

By magic? – life is full, with four children, coaching rugby and practising yoga everyday – try to fill up the jar!

My ambitions for the future

Always 'save the world'! – perhaps more realistically (and seriously), I work as a servant to the public – I still want to make a tangible difference to people's health and wellbeing, and so to their lives. Increasingly, I think this is about redressing inequity (unfair differences) in health and life chances – I aspire to making a contribution to reducing inequity, and helping others in public service do that too, through their work.

My advice to the next generation

'None of us knows as much as all of us …', and 'win or learn' – so be humble and ask.

Yeyenta Osasu, National Pharmacy Integration Lead, NHS England

Developing an early interest in public health

As a young girl, growing up in a tropical environment, I was aware of several infectious diseases and interested in knowing how the human body functioned, why people got sick and why we feel pain. I was interested to know how medication alleviates pain – how did the medicine know the exact part of the body to work on and how did it get there? These questions swirled through my mind, and I was often perplexed at all the questions a doctor would ask me or my mother whenever I was poorly. My inquisitive mind wanted to understand why I was being asked such questions and how my answers influenced the doctor's decisions. Sometimes, I would offer incorrect answers to doctors' questions to test if they would work out the missing piece of the puzzle, come to the right conclusion and offer the right treatment. I was inquisitive!

I realised in my teenage years that I liked chemistry and biology, particularly because these pure science subjects provided answers to my curious mind and I began to understand how, and why, things worked. I was also interested in geography and social studies because I was curious about people, cultures and the environment. These personal interests influenced my choice of subjects for A-Level exams and subsequent first degree in pharmacy.

While studying at university, I enjoyed courses such as medicinal chemistry and pharmacology, but was deeply fascinated about the social determinants of health and the inequities that resulted in poorer health outcomes for some.

Getting started on a career in public health pharmacy, training and experience

Prior to my university degree, I worked in a pharmacy at weekends as a pharmacy counter assistant and enjoyed speaking to different people. I offered medication counselling and suggested treatment for minor ailments with over-the-counter medicines, for which I had taken the appropriate training. Following this, I studied pharmacy at the School of Pharmacy, University College London, and obtained a Master's degree in Pharmacy.

I started my career as a junior pharmacist working in mental health at St. Charles Hospital, Central and North West London NHS Foundation Trust, South London and Maudsley NHS Foundation Trust and St. Ann's Hospital, London. Following these early roles, I progressed to Senior Clinical Pharmacist at Chesterfield Royal Hospital, where I worked as an anticoagulation pharmacist.

As I progressed in my career, I obtained further qualifications and training, including a Post-graduate Diploma in Clinical Pharmacy and an Independent Prescribing qualification. I undertook the Mary Seacole Leadership programme, obtained a PhD in medicines optimisation and was successfully selected as a national population health fellow.

While I found clinical pharmacy interesting, I knew that I wanted to broaden my experience, so I took advantage of a population health fellowship opportunity with Health Education England. The experience I gained during the fellowship year was interesting and different from anything I had done before in healthcare.

Public health roles

Working in primary care within GP surgeries as a practice pharmacist with Derby and Derbyshire Clinical Commissioning Group (CCG) brought me closer to understanding the way in which social determinants of health influenced health outcomes. My secondment to Health Education England (HEE) and working with the Director of Public Health (DPH) at a local City Council provided me the opportunity to work on health improvement and prevention projects during the COVID-19 pandemic.

My public health contribution during the pandemic

I was involved in three key public health projects during the pandemic:

- I developed a medicines delivery service for clinically vulnerable individuals;
- I designed and developed materials to support clinically vulnerable individuals maintain physical activity during lockdown; and
- I co-developed and worked on a local strategy for addressing health inequalities through the COVID-19 vaccine roll-out programme, including engaging with members of local communities to address vaccine hesitancy.

Below is an example of my contribution to key public health issues stemming from the pandemic:

A Report of the Medicines Delivery Service in Sheffield during the COVID-19 Pandemic

Introduction

This report summarises the work undertaken to organise community action to support vulnerable and shielding individuals across Sheffield in accessing their medication following the lockdown during the COVID-19 pandemic.

Background

The UK government introduced public health guidance and stringent lockdown measures following the outbreak of COVID-19. Some people who were particularly susceptible to poor outcomes following coronavirus infection were identified as clinically vulnerable and advised to take particular care to minimise contact with others outside their household. A further group of people with serious health conditions were advised to adopt shielding measures to keep themselves safe by staying at home and avoiding all contact with others, except for essential medical treatment or support. This group of people, who are more likely to have multiple health conditions, were at increased risk of social isolation and would have been unable to obtain their medication from the community pharmacy, as the pharmacies were also under considerable pressure during this time. This meant that pharmacies that would normally deliver medication to patients were struggling to keep up with rising demand from members of the public as their staff and delivery drivers began to self-isolate due to the pandemic.

This project was designed to ensure that vulnerable patients who relied on essential medicines could still access their medication without the risk of exposure to Coronavirus infection.

What we did

We worked collaboratively to support people with serious health conditions in Sheffield to receive their medication while shielding. This involved, firstly, speaking to two local community pharmacies to understand if there was a need to support them in delivering medicines to patients, and how the COVID-19 pandemic affected their daily workload. The need to support pharmacies to continue medication deliveries was immediately identified.

Secondly, the population health pharmacist set up a group of volunteers to support vulnerable people and community pharmacies by undertaking a number of duties, which included delivering readymade medication packages to the homes of these individuals, taking people to and from appointments at the hospital or pharmacy, and helping community pharmacies with daily administrative tasks.

The Medication Delivery Service

A group of 45 core volunteers were identified and recruited. This initial group were provided with guidance documents on how to handle and deliver medications safely to the right individuals. They were supported with up-to-date guidance from Public Health England on maintaining a safe distance, and the necessary hygiene measures that were required to keep them and others safe. Volunteers were also provided with documents to read which improved their confidence in handling medicines.

The population health pharmacist worked closely with council-based community support workers at the central hub and received referrals concerning individuals who required medication pick up from pharmacies and delivery to people's homes. Upon receiving the referrals, a call would be put out to volunteers through a secure digital platform, stating the area of the city and the job required, without disclosing any identifiable personal information. Available volunteers responded promptly, and the job was assigned and confirmed over the telephone. The staff at the central hub were notified when each task was assigned and completed.

The service was coordinated solely by the population health pharmacist from 26 March until 9 April 2020, when staff from the Clinical Commissioning Group (CCG) were assigned to assist with coordination of the Volunteers as the need for the service expanded. The CCG staff and two University of Sheffield medical students assisted in coordinating volunteers from 9 April to 18 May 2020. The population health pharmacist continued to provide support to the volunteer coordinators through the process. Subsequently, collaborative networks were made with stakeholders, including Voluntary Action Sheffield and Sheffield Accountable Care Partnership.

As time elapsed and the lockdown continued in varying forms, working circumstances also evolved. It soon became necessary to coordinate volunteers more centrally as the service grew and developed. The medication delivery service also evolved, and the volunteers registered with Voluntary Action Sheffield, where they continued to provide support locally.

Subsequent public health roles

The COVID-19 pandemic highlighted the inequalities that existed prior to the pandemic and the NHS responded by ensuring that efforts were made to reduce inequities in healthcare access and delivery, particularly in some demographic groups. After the population health fellowship, I took on a new role as Regional Health Equity Improvement Manager.

Some of my duties included acting as an ambassador for health equity improvement across the health and care sector, advocating the rights of potentially disadvantaged and marginalised communities, all of which provided an opportunity to challenge existing or proposed new practices within a range of different forums.

This exciting role gave me the opportunity to work across systems and sectors. I met with, and developed, work streams with various people at very senior levels within organisations and I enjoyed influencing policy in a meaningful way that positively affected how some groups of people accessed, experienced and received care within health and social care settings.

In my current role as National Pharmacy Integration Lead at NHS England, I lead on the Community Pharmacy Hypertension Case Finding Service, where I work strategically with several national stakeholders and patients to improve the diagnosis of hypertension in people who would otherwise not have known that they have a raised blood pressure. This role has given me the opportunity to put clinical and population health skills into practice, while reducing health inequalities and improving access to healthcare.

Maintaining a work/life balance

Working in public health during a pandemic has meant working long hours, mostly at home, and attending online meetings much more than usual. I have tried to manage this by ensuring that I take regular rest breaks and a half-hour walk during the day. This latter gives me the opportunity to clear my head while taking in some fresh air and vitamin D through natural sunlight. Consequently, I get rewarded with a burst of energy and new ideas for the rest of my working day.

My ambitions for the future

As I progress in my career, I hope to continue developing and strengthening my use of data intelligence to inform the work that I do and to engage with people at a broader level. I also hope to improve health at a population level and to play a major part in improving health literacy and providing value to communities in a way that reduces disease burden and prevents ill health.

My advice to the next generation

While some future and aspiring public health professionals may consider applying for a Master's in Public Health (MPH) programme, a more accessible place to start could involve engaging in volunteering opportunities in local voluntary and charity organisations. This provides the benefit of understanding the daily challenges faced by people and how social circumstances, including finance, affect health and wellbeing. Work collaboratively across teams and it is usually helpful to gain experience in unfamiliar areas. It is also helpful to work inclusively and seek opportunities to meet and speak to people whom you may not usually spend time with. This has the advantage of broadening perspectives and developing equitable, culturally competent and trauma-informed approaches to health and social care delivery.

Notes

  i A place-based approach is about understanding the issues, interconnections and relationships in a place and coordinating action and investment to improve the quality of life for that community.

  ii Non-governmental and non-profit-making organisations or associations, including charities, voluntary and community groups, cooperatives, etc.

iii See Part 4.

References

1. Scottish Government. *Improving Public Services*. Available at: www.gov.scot/policies/improving-public-services/community-planning/.
2. Davies, S.C., Winpenny, E., Ball, S., Fowler, T., Rubin R. and Nolte, E. For debate: A new wave in health improvement. *The Lancet*, 3 April 2014. Available at: www.thelancet.com/journals/lancet/article/PIIS0140-6736(13)62341-7/fulltext.
3. West, R. and Gould, A. *WHO Collaborating Centre on Investment for Health and Wellbeing*. Available at: https://phwwhocc.co.uk/resources/improving-health-and-wellbeing-a-guide-to-using-behavioural-science-in-policy-and-practice.

3 Health intelligence

The centrality of information

Myer Glickman; John Battersby;
Matt Hennessey; Natalie Adams; Fiona Sim;
Jenny Wright

Introduction to this function

Health intelligence practitioners and specialists collect, analyse, interpret and communicate information about health. This information may be drawn from data about the general health and wellbeing of a specified population, or about the health risks and health needs of a particular group within society (such as an age group or an ethnic group or people with a particular medical condition). The role is critical in supporting decision-makers across the health and healthcare system to understand the needs of the population, and to identify risks and priorities for action, by converting raw data from many different sources into meaningful information about health and wellbeing to be used by a largely non-specialist audience, such as councillors and council staff, hospital trusts, commissioners and government, as well as the general public.

During the pandemic, health intelligence specialists and practitioners proved vital in keeping the public and policy makers informed of the latest anonymised data relating to the pandemic, including numbers of cases, numbers in hospital, numbers who were discharged from hospital and numbers who sadly died, as well as, later in the pandemic, those vaccinated – health data and epidemiology have never been so popular. They were also essential in providing information on changes in other indicators of health and wellbeing in the population during the pandemic.

Future challenges and opportunities – a vision for health intelligence

Myer Glickman, Head of Epidemiology, Climate and
Global Health, Office for National Statistics

Public health intelligence – the systematic collection and analysis of information about health risks, impacts and outcomes – is both an integral part of public health from its earliest days and an exciting field at the cutting edge of science. The history of public health is a story of statistical tables like the London Bills of Mortality,[1] charts such as William Farr's epidemic curve,[2] maps such as those by John Snow on cholera[3] and innovative data

DOI: 10.4324/9781003433699-5

visualisations from Florence Nightingale's polar charts onwards.[4] The future points in many directions – real-time monitoring of health trends to inform urgent decisions, data exploration at increasingly precise local resolutions, synthesis of wide-ranging data to better describe the complex influences on our lives and health, and tools to exploit the potential of 'big data'.

The COVID-19 pandemic brought public health intelligence very much into the limelight. Systems and processes were stress-tested, revealing simultaneously strengths and weaknesses, exciting possibilities and frustrating bottlenecks. One lesson that came through very quickly was that modern government needs a lot of data, and it needs it fast! That means traditional timescales like annual or quarterly reports are just no good in an emergency. For the institutions of official statistics, one crucial theme was the need to think more creatively about speed of reporting, while maintaining reliability of the figures.

Another lesson that became obvious was that government and NHS organisations are mostly bad at sharing and exploiting their huge stocks of data efficiently, a systemic problem born of multiple legal and policy frameworks and institutional fragmentation. But despite that, innovative linked databases were built and new methods made a real impact on understanding pandemic and health issues beyond. Some surprising applications of data science moved into the realms of real application, like testing for COVID-19 variants in sewage.[5]

Just as the pandemic highlighted existing social and health inequalities, it also shone more light on existing aspects of public health intelligence. The need for more joined-up data and analysis across geographies and institutions was nothing new. Lack of consistent health intelligence structures and resources across local government was already a known problem, and smaller teams were stretched even further by the urgent needs of local services and decision-makers. But the importance of health intelligence became obvious to the whole nation in a way it never has before, bringing new potential to the field.

The changes we are likely to see in future are ones that will make public health intelligence an ever-more fascinating career. The fast-moving world of data science means there will constantly be new skills to learn, and new opportunities for those with aptitude and enthusiasm. Emerging sub-specialties like data engineering provide more diversity of job openings for the technically minded, while the power of R, Python and whatever language comes next allows the production of complex analyses and revealing visualisations more quickly and easily than in the past. Analysts can expect to work with larger, more integrated multi-source datasets that have more power to answer both old and new public health questions.

Greater recognition of the interdependency of organisations and disciplines to tackle public health problems at all levels – local, national and global – should open up more opportunities for those specialising in the field to learn from one another and progress through a wider range of career paths. A major innovation in training is a new Health and Care Intelligence Specialist apprenticeship pathway in England.[i] At the same time, public health intelligence will doubtless continue to be strengthened by drawing in talented people from many different backgrounds.

Overview of the health intelligence function

John Battersby, Consultant in Public Health, Public Health Analysis Unit, Office for Health Improvement and Disparities (OHID)

What is health intelligence?

Health intelligence involves the collection, analysis, interpretation and communication of information about the health of populations or groups within a population. Health intelligence sometimes gets called public health analysis, or health information, but these refer to the same set of activities.

People working in health intelligence have a variety of job titles, such as public health analyst, intelligence officer, data scientist, information officer, knowledge facilitator, registration officer and so on. They can be found working in various settings, including the private and charitable sectors, as well as the more usual public sector organisations.

Why health intelligence is important

Understanding how any complex system works inevitably requires lots of data and information. The pilot of an aircraft needs to know how fast and how high they are flying, how well their engines are functioning, the status of various pieces of equipment, etc. Similarly, governments need to understand the health of their populations so that they can allocate resources to where the need is greatest and decide which policies to pursue. At a more local level, councils and hospitals need to understand the health of the populations they serve so that they can ensure that appropriate services are provided to the right people.

A good example of this is the response to the COVID-19 pandemic which, at all levels, relied on accurate and up-to-date information about the numbers of people testing positive, the number going into hospital and so on. Public health intelligence analysts made a major contribution to the COVID-19 response through their work analysing data, developing dashboards[6] and providing a wide variety of essential information to help inform evidence-based policies for issues such as school closures. It is through the work of people in health intelligence that we understand which groups in the population have poorer health or health outcomes. Work to address inequalities in health relies on accurate information about the nature of the inequalities that are experienced. Health intelligence analysts will look at information about risk factors or behaviours that influence ill-health, such as smoking, or physical activity, and analyse it to understand differences by age, gender, income, geography, ethnicity and other relevant factors. They will do similar types of analyses on data about diseases to understand the patterns and variations in those diseases, whether there are inequalities in the amount of disease or the disease outcomes, and which groups within the population are most affected by those inequalities.

Some health intelligence work focuses on diseases which can be transmitted from one person or species to another. These are known as communicable diseases and include common infections such as COVID-19 and influenza, as well as less common infections such as diphtheria and measles. Other teams focus more on non-communicable diseases, such as heart disease, diabetes and mental health conditions. However, the pandemic has demonstrated the interrelationship between these groups of diseases and there are examples of analytical work that seek to shed light on the wider impacts of diseases such as COVID. The Wider Impact of COVID-19 on Health (WICH) tool is a good example of this.[7]

Analysts in health intelligence roles also work with data which are generated by the health and care system. For example, understanding how patients move through the health system, from when they see their GP through to leaving hospital, having received the appropriate treatment. This is essential for making improvements to the care received by those patients.

Roles for health intelligence analysts

Health intelligence roles can be found in a broad range of organisations and the roles themselves can be very varied. The importance of health intelligence in underpinning public health work means that most organisations that employ public health staff will include health intelligence staff among them. In England, the main organisations that have public health roles are the national organisations such as the UK Health Security Agency (UKHSA) and the Office for Health Improvement and Disparities (OHID) and, at a more local level, unitary, county and borough councils. These probably employ most people in public health intelligence, but there are many other organisations that employ smaller numbers, including:

- commissioning organisations, such as Integrated Care Systems;
- NHS Hospital or Community Trusts;
- academic settings, such as universities with research teams;
- health charities; and
- the private sector.

One of the great things about health intelligence is that it offers such a variety of opportunities. Although many roles are analytical in nature, there is increasing demand in health intelligence teams to bring in data scientists and software developers. Interpreting and translating health information for decision-makers is another important aspect of health intelligence work and there is always a need for people with good communication and knowledge translation skills.

What makes a good health intelligence analyst?

People who work in health intelligence need to be comfortable handling data, particularly data in the form of numbers. A good understanding of maths or statistics is particularly helpful, but many people come into health intelligence having studied subjects such as geography, psychology or biology.

As well as people who are good with numbers, health intelligence teams include people with skills in web and app development – particularly, skills in data science (handling very large datasets using computer programming approaches). This is because the way that health intelligence analysts work has changed markedly over the last few years. Instead of using spreadsheets, analysts often use coding approaches, where analytical software can be programmed to download data, analyse it and produce a report which is then sent out automatically. Programming languages that are frequently used are R and Python.

There is an increased use of online dashboards for data and indicators. These require analysts to ensure that the data are analysed correctly, as well as software developers to develop the dashboard itself. Another development has been the use of apps on mobile devices that can collect useful data, which can then be analysed for both the app user and for health planners. Examples of this are collecting data on keywords from social media platforms like Twitter to provide warning of disease outbreaks and apps like *Couch to 5K* to help people become more active.[8]

Many people enter health intelligence roles early in their career and then move up to more senior roles as they gain experience. Others move in from analytical roles in other business sectors. There are also a small number of health intelligence roles for public health specialists and these are often of interest to people who have experience of analytical work, either before they entered public health training or from placements they did while training.

Starting off in health intelligence

It can be difficult to get into a health intelligence role before you have much experience. Fortunately, that is starting to change. There are now several apprenticeship standards in data analysis and data science and employers of health intelligence staff are using these to recruit into health intelligence roles. These allow you to study for a further qualification while working as an analyst. The apprenticeship standards which are suitable for people wishing to follow a career in health intelligence are available to both school leavers and graduates.

If you are keen to start a career in health intelligence, anything that gives you experience of handling and analysing data is useful. This could be through school or college projects or perhaps through work experience in an analytical role; even if it is not health-based, it will nevertheless provide good experience.

Graduates in subjects such as maths, statistics and computer science should find themselves well placed to find suitable roles and some organisations have graduate entry schemes for health analysts.

Health intelligence makes a difference

Although it is easy to think of health intelligence as a 'back office' or supporting activity, it is the work of the health intelligence community that drives much of the work to improve population health. Two examples might help to illustrate this further:

The first is taken from work that was completed across a local area in South East England. Data about the risk factors for diabetes and the people within the population that had particular risk factors were linked with geographical data that allowed public health staff to predict where in their community they were most likely to find people with a high risk of developing diabetes, or with undiagnosed diabetes. This allowed them to put in place interventions to both help people to address their risk of developing diabetes and for healthcare workers to identify people within these particular communities that had already developed diabetes so that they could benefit from treatment.

The second example is the national work that has been done to provide both the public and policy makers with accurate and timely information about the COVID-19 pandemic. A team of health intelligence analysts, data scientists and software developers worked together to develop England's national COVID-19 dashboard. This brought together dozens of complex data flows to produce clear and accurate information on the progress of the pandemic. The dashboard has grown to the point at which, in 2022, it had around two million users every week. It has developed to include dynamic maps, as well as charts, and the data are downloadable for others to analyse.

My journey into health intelligence

My own interest in health intelligence started before I entered public health. At the time I was overseeing a primary care project in a rural area of Tunisia. It was important that I and the rest of the project team understood what the main health problems were in the area where we worked and that we were able to collect relevant data to help us evaluate the impact of our work. To help lead that work, I was fortunate enough to be sent on a short course in epidemiology and statistics at the London School of Hygiene and Tropical Medicine (LSHTM), where I learned about carrying out surveys and analysing the results. I was able to use that knowledge back on the ground in Tunisia and share it with others.

When I returned from Tunisia, I entered training as a specialist in public health. I was able to continue my interest in health intelligence through a training placement at one of the regional public health observatories which had been set up to monitor the health of the populations they covered. On completing training, I worked as a Director of Public Health (DPH), so was very much a user of health intelligence. I worked closely with health intelligence colleagues to produce profiles of our populations and health needs assessments that allowed us to commission appropriate services for our population of around one million.

After around six years as a DPH, a job was advertised back in the Public Health Observatory and it was a natural progression for me to apply for it. I found myself leading the observatory's analytical team, doing some 'hands on' analytical work and overseeing a project to develop a new set of profiles which presented health information about GP practices across England.[9]

I have remained in health intelligence since then and enjoyed various roles and always been mindful of the opportunity that I have had to influence health decisions using good quality data and information. Most recently, my role has concentrated on developing skills within the analytical workforce, especially the coding and programming skills mentioned earlier, and developing the Health and Care Intelligence Specialist apprenticeship standards. It has been very rewarding, and unusually for a public health role, has let me see a rapid change in the way that analytical work is done and the impact this has had on the range of health intelligence products that are produced. The response to the COVID-19 pandemic has particularly drawn on the skills of the health intelligence community and has been an excellent example of 'data-driven decisions'.

Career stories

Matt Hennessey, Chief Intelligence and Analytics Officer for NHS Greater Manchester Integrated Care

Introduction

Reflecting on my career to date for this chapter, I realised that for as long as I have been in full-time employment – which is now nearly 25 years – I have been working in the field of public health. You wouldn't necessarily know that from my CV though. The only time the words 'Public Health' appear in any of my job titles during my career is a short period of about one year and one month in 2013. The list of qualifications in my CV doesn't give much away either, because there's nothing there that overtly indicates any formal public health training. So perhaps I'm an unusual choice to be asked to contribute to a book on public health careers. However, despite being apparently underqualified on paper to contribute to a discussion of public health careers, I have spent my career and certainly every single day of the last 15 years working directly with public health practitioners, specialists, consultants and directors at local, regional and national levels. So how does someone get to spend so much time working in the field of public health without becoming 'labelled' a public health professional? The answer (for some people) is when you work in data, analytics and intelligence.

Getting started on a public health career

Clearly, I did not set out on a public health career path, but neither did I set out to work in health intelligence. My first degree was in psychology and my career aspirations, such as they were at that time, revolved around becoming either a clinical or forensic psychologist. My early career considerations coincided with a general increase in the public interest of criminal psychology following some high-profile murder cases and Jimmy McGovern's TV series 'Cracker'. Cultural and contemporary influences have shaped a significant proportion of my career and the COVID-19 pandemic will undoubtedly have a similar impact on students exploring careers in public health, epidemiology, virology and health intelligence.

Experience of working in a forensic setting was a prerequisite to securing a place on a post-graduate qualification course and career in forensic psychology, and my first exposure to public health came when I successfully applied to be a Probation Service Officer with Merseyside Probation Service. I was placed with the Substance Misuse Team and deployed to Wirral Drug Service based at St. Catherine's Hospital. If you want to be exposed to the real value of public health and the consequences of inadequate public policy, then there is truly no more educative experience than working with substance misuser/addicted offenders. Individual choices and personal responsibility are, of course, a fundamental part of offending and addiction, but the influences of a negative environment were so manifest that they could have been lifted straight from the pages of Professor Sir Michael Marmot's seminal work, The Health Gap.[10] Marmot asks: 'Why treat people and send them back to the conditions that make them sick?' and, in my work with the drug service, I saw childhood trauma, poor housing, unfulfilled academic potential, unemployment, domestic abuse, malnutrition and the inter-relationship with poor physical and mental health through co-morbidity, communicable disease and a learned lack of personal agency.

Training and gaining experience

As a substance misuse and probation worker, there was a large amount of mandatory training. This was training that you would also expect to see on a public health curriculum – risk assessment, safeguarding, communicable disease and blood-borne viruses, domestic abuse, motivational interviewing, clinical practice and personal development, change management and the law. Armed with this training and a couple of years' front-line experience in a variety of different forensic settings, I secured a role as a trainee forensic psychologist with the Prison Service. On account of my substance misuse experience and unusually for such a role, I was posted to the Area Office, where my role was to work with the 16 prison establishments in the North West to develop drug strategies and evidence-based substance misuse interventions. The Forensic Psychology curriculum, much like that of public health, had both operational and strategic components exploring roles as both practitioners and leaders.

Moving into public health roles

Over time, I became increasingly involved in the strategy work and subsequently moved to a role at the Home Office leading drug and alcohol strategy for the North West region. Machinery of government changes are a constant feature of public sector working and although I retained a specialism in substance misuse, the formation of the Office of the Deputy Prime Minister and Government Offices meant that new policy initiatives were frequently tacked on to the main job and for me these included community cohesion, preventing violent extremism and place-based responsibilities for negotiating delivery targets with local government – known as Local Area Agreements.[11] These latter three activities provided wide exposure to the totality of community and place-based activity. Having to negotiate targets to help reduce traffic congestion, crime and health inequalities, as well as help increase economic output, educational attainment and decent housing, was a lesson in the complexity of public policy interaction. This was also the first time I was asked to really flex any analytical muscles I had – modelling proposed delivery targets and potential stretch targets against financial incentives. Working at the Government Office in the region meant I was also frequently drawn into emergency planning exercises and contributed to regional resilience committees.

In 2008, I was appointed Joint Head of the Alcohol Harm Reduction National Support Team at the Department of Health. The Public Health National Support Teams (NSTs) were established to provide 'consultancy-style support and assistance to local health economies across England'.[12] The Alcohol NST team conducted 34-week-long local authority visits over the course of two-and-a-half years.[13] In this role, I was presented with the opportunity to see how public health was perceived and implemented in different areas right across the country and engage with public health leaders at every level, from Government Ministers to front-line practitioners. I also found myself spending more time working with data and intelligence – trying to understand more about what sat behind an area's public health challenges and working out how to evaluate the impact and effectiveness of their efforts to improve things. As any textbook about public health will attest, some public health interventions can take years or even decades to realise their full benefits. It is a source of constant frustration in a world that demands 'quick wins', so the value in being able to make the business case for public health investment was becoming ever-more important. Ironically, the NSTs themselves fell victim to the timeliness of returns on public health investment and the programme did not survive the austerity measures that were introduced following the banking crisis, but a recent evaluation of the Health Inequalities Strategy, of which the NSTs were part, found the programme had a positive impact.[14]

The combination of training and experience in the individual components of public health over many years resulted in my being appointed a Fellow of the Royal Society for Public Health. I thought long and hard about trying to consolidate my public health experience in some form of specialist qualification (such as Master in Public Health), but feeling that my experience spoke for itself, I opted to study for a Master of Business Administration (MBA) in Executive Leadership, which I obtained in 2014. I became increasingly interested in how data and intelligence could support leadership decision-making and public health ambitions,[15] and this led to a more focused health intelligence career path, beginning with a role leading public health intelligence at the North West Public Health Observatory (NWPHO), and then as Associate Director of Local Knowledge and Intelligence Services (North West) within Health Intelligence Division of Public Health England (PHE).[ii]

My contribution to public health

A key feature of my career journey has been how my career horizon has always been towards the medium rather than long term. This means that my knowledge and skills have always been heavily shaped by the employment environment of any given moment. Working at NWPHO and PHE and in close proximity to data and analysis experts in public service and, in particular, within academia, has provided me with exposure to the very latest advancements in technology and statistical methodologies, and I've come to appreciate that the unique contribution I can make, given the broad public sector experience I have, is to connect the highly technical work of analysts to those who can benefit from it. Since 2019, I have been the Chief Intelligence and Analytics Officer at the Greater Manchester Health and Social Care Partnership (which is now called NHS Greater Manchester) and my role has been to do exactly that – support leaders and key decision-makers to understand what intelligence they require and mobilise the technical expertise to provide it. The most satisfying thing about this role and working in health intelligence and, in particular, public health intelligence, is a feeling that you are part of the glue that connects all aspects of public policy. As stakeholders right across the system come to recognise the importance of intelligence-informed decision making, they are increasingly relying on public health analysts to provide a holistic assessment of system impact, which means working with all stakeholders.

The impact of the pandemic on health intelligence workload and maintaining a work/life balance

Health intelligence has undergone a renaissance as a result of the pandemic, as indeed has public health generally. *The New York Times* declared 'epidemiologists to be the new rock stars'.[16] If that is the case, then we data geeks are surely the new energy magnates. Data, like energy, has become an indispensable commodity, the true value of which has only recently started to be realised among the wider population and those who do not deal with it on a daily basis. There was a time when I would have scoffed at the idea that a data analyst might need to be 'on call', but not anymore. Intelligence has been thrust right into the frontline of emergency planning and is rightfully respected for the value it can bring to a variety of strategic and operational situations. However, dealing with this newfound popularity can be a challenge, since for many analysts the attraction of solving complex problems and staying on top of rapid technology innovation isn't just a job, it's also a hobby, and so maintaining a healthy work/life balance and stepping away from the computer screen and the tech is vitally important. I'm not sure it is a balance I have fully mastered yet, but through a combination of volunteering in my local community woodland and taking up some yoga and meditation practice, I am hoping to both keep active and fit and also make time to be more 'present' and less analytical.

Why health intelligence is a rewarding career

With this renewed interest in what health intelligence provides comes a resurgence in its appeal as a career, but navigating the health intelligence and public health intelligence landscape is tricky. Health intelligence – like public health – requires a combination of many disciplines and skills. The technological advances that have occurred in cloud computing and data management coupled with new data science and statistical techniques now demand a new breed of analyst. The first challenge to overcome is understanding what you are pursuing a career in. Data Science? Informatics? Data engineering? Data analysis? Data Evangelist? The government has produced a useful profession capability framework which describes some of these emerging digital, data and technology roles.[17]

Being part of a new movement that embraces the full capability of new technologies, analytics and advances in statistical thinking is genuinely exciting. Galvanised by a newfound appreciation of the value of data and analytics, intelligence community members are coming together in a much more coordinated way. AnalystX, an NHS England-facilitated community of interest, now has thousands of members and there is an emerging professionalism which will support workforce and career development.[18]

My career journey into public health intelligence always felt like the exception rather than the rule, but I've come to realise that health intelligence is a path that most analysts working today inadvertently found while on a journey somewhere else. However, by accident or by design, a career in health intelligence is a rewarding one. Speak to anyone working in this field and you will find they belong to a community that is passionate about their work, values neurodiversity and is inclusive, and where job satisfaction is high.[19] Unlike for other established occupations in areas such as medicine, accountancy or law, there has never been the same big door advertising 'this way for a career in health intelligence'. I hope, and believe, this will change as a greater professionalism and emphasis on workforce development, coupled with a newfound admiration for the role of the data analyst, will start to influence early career conversations.

In 2018, it was estimated that 2.5 quadrillion bytes of new data were created every single day and in 2020 the number of bytes in the digital universe was 40 times bigger than the number of stars in the observable universe.[20] In an uncertain world, one thing we can be pretty sure of is that there's going to be no shortage of work for the future analysts to do!

Natalie Adams, Public Health Intelligence Practitioner
and Specialty Registrar in Public Health

My start in public health

I started my journey in health intelligence via a geography project at school exploring the spatial epidemiology of malaria. The challenges of identifying reliable data to map malaria cases across different countries sparked my longstanding interest in the field of public health and the use of data to inform, and provide context for, important epidemiological questions.

I see health intelligence as a cornerstone of public health practice; integral to enabling us to move from data to decisions. This is often described as the 'data-to-decision journey' and this is something I always try to keep in mind when I am seeking to combine data and evidence to help inform decision making at any level.

At the time I was considering my career and university options in 2005–2006, there were very limited options to study epidemiology or public health at undergraduate level in the UK. Now, many universities offer specific degrees in both, as well as many module options. I started university in 2007 and chose the University of Nottingham's School of Geography, as they offered modules in medical geography. Although perhaps not an obvious choice for someone interested in a career in health intelligence or epidemiology, the skills I gained in my Geography degree equipped me with an understanding of statistics, Geographic Information System (GIS) mapping, politics, sanitation, health inequalities and the wider determinants of health. Knowing I wanted a career in public health, I was able to focus on an epidemiological question for my dissertation: exploring the statistical and spatial relationship between Encephalitis Lethargica and Scarlet Fever in England and Wales in the 1920s. After emailing medical archives across the country to find out where the relevant records were held, I managed to spend an exciting summer delving through historical health records at various archives, including at the Wellcome Collection in London and Nottinghamshire archives.

Nottingham University also had a fantastic internal internship programme whereby students could apply to work on discrete projects over the summer. This gave the students experience of academic research, as well as exposure to interviews and recruitment, as the internships were a competitive application process. I spent two summers working on projects, including qualitative research into attitudes of overweight and obesity, as well as developing mobile applications to support the administration of questionnaires to investigate gastrointestinal infections.

Gaining experience in public health and further academic work

It was at this time that I first learned about the Public Health Specialty Training Scheme via one of my Geography lecturers, and so I decided to remain in Nottingham to complete a Master's in Public Health. In the summer prior to starting my Master's, and following on from the contacts I made in the internship exploring mobile applications for gastrointestinal infection outbreaks, I was invited to undertake work experience with the national gastrointestinal infections team at the Health Protection Agency (now the UK Health Security Agency (UKHSA)) for a two-week placement. Although very short, it was an excellent insight into the practical application of epidemiology and gave me good grounding for my Master's. Throughout my Master's, I retained a strong interest in the use of health data to inform public health decisions, selecting modules focused on epidemiology and statistics.

After my Master's, I set about searching for jobs, and while the job market at the time for public health graduates was small, I was ultimately successful in securing a role as an epidemiologist in the same department of the Health Protection Agency I had completed my work experience in over two years earlier. In this role, I worked primarily on the national surveillance of gastrointestinal pathogens, such as norovirus, rotavirus, Shiga-toxin producing *E. coli* (STEC) and national foodborne and non-foodborne outbreaks. The importance of understanding the strengths and limitations of the underlying data and ensuring the quality of that data and subsequent analyses to enable effective decisions was evident on a daily basis in the almost seven years I spent in this role. This was especially the case when investigating outbreaks: the need to ensure accuracy and precision at every stage from data collection and entry through to statistical analysis was paramount to correctly identifying the source of the outbreak and ultimately implementing public health action to prevent further illness.

A few years into this role, the opportunity arose to apply for a PhD as part of the first National Institute for Health and Care Research (NIHR) Health Protection Research Unit in Gastrointestinal Infections in conjunction with the University of Liverpool, as well as the Universities of Oxford and East Anglia. I was excited by the prospect of being able to combine my background in epidemiology and the social determinants of health with my interest in applied academic research, and I could see a direct link between the research and the day-to-day surveillance work of the gastrointestinal infections department at Public Health England (PHE). As part of this, I completed a PhD exploring socioeconomic inequalities in risk of and exposure to gastrointestinal infections in the UK. The aim of this PhD was to better understand inequalities in risk and exposure at different points of the surveillance pyramid, attempting to account for the potential for inequalities in whether people seek medical help for their symptoms and in what capacity they do so. I undertook analyses on several large datasets, including NHS Direct (online medical advice service[iii]) and NHS 111 (out-of-hours' primary medical care telephone advice service), which enabled me to gain experience of using different data linkage techniques and explore analyses in different statistical software packages. It was a great opportunity to utilise existing surveillance datasets and generate insights that fed directly into policy and practice.

After completing my PhD, I wanted to seek experience in health intelligence within a local authority to broaden my understanding of this aspect of public health at a local rather than national level. I became the Senior Public Health Intelligence Specialist for the London Borough of Bexley, and spent a year working on developing health intelligence systems including local dashboards and supporting health needs assessments. I was in this role when COVID-19 first emerged. In the initial weeks after COVID-19 was identified and then declared as a pandemic, there was a real need to try and understand the possible impacts on the local area, including estimates of cases, hospitalisations and deaths against a background of uncertainty about severity and infectiousness. There was also a need to develop processes rapidly to collate data and intelligence on the actual impacts in as close to real-time as possible, while acting within the legal frameworks for data sharing and a constantly changing picture of the gravity of the situation. While national data gave an important overview of the situation, the need for timely data at a local level was evident from the beginning and it was important to ensure information was presented in a balanced way, with clear caveats and limitations, to assist with decision making and targeted local action. For me, the pandemic typifies the importance of both quantitative and qualitative data within public health. The data, coupled with high-quality public health intelligence, complements the work of local authority teams by providing the evidence base for a wide range of public health action.

Joining the higher specialist training scheme

The desire to join the Public Health Training Scheme had not diminished over this time and I finally felt that the time was right to apply, having gained some experience in national and local public health. The application process consists of an initial application form followed by a series of assessments, details of which, as well as eligibility criteria, are included on the Faculty of Public Health website.[iv, 21]

I started my current role as a Public Health Specialty Registrar in August 2020. The training scheme is an excellent opportunity for anyone interested in becoming a Consultant in Public Health: it is a four- to five-year programme during which time you undertake placements in different organisations to gain experience of the different aspects of public health you might encounter, or specialise in, as a future leader. To date, I have completed placements in a local authority public health team, as well as in local Health Protection and in academia, contributing to COVID-19 research and surveillance. I am hoping that I will be able to retain an emphasis on and interest in health intelligence throughout my career, even when it may not be the obvious focus of my role.

Why I find health intelligence rewarding

Health intelligence is both challenging and rewarding. It is incredibly satisfying to provide insights that directly contribute to evidence-based decisions being made. It also requires you to constantly seek to evolve your skillset to rise to the challenge of answering new and often difficult questions. I am passionate about embedding health intelligence in all aspects of public health, as I believe it has a crucial role in facilitating the data-to-decision journey. I think all those working in public health have a duty to understand the importance of health intelligence, even if it is not their area of specialism, and for those of us who have a passion for health intelligence, I also believe it is our duty to make it as accessible for others as we can.

My advice to the next generation

My top five tips for anyone interested in health intelligence are to:

- think broadly – so many experiences are applicable to public health practice;
- seize every opportunity you can to further your knowledge and skills, including networking and identifying relevant conferences or seminars you can attend;
- consider the 'so what' when generating and explaining information to ensure the data-to-decision journey is at the forefront of your work;
- be curious – ask lots of questions and speak to as many people as you can about your work and theirs; and
- be clear about what the data or information *is* telling you as well as what it is *not*.

Notes

i See the overview and the section on undergraduate education in Part 4 for details of this scheme.
ii NWPHO, which was hosted at Liverpool John Moores University, became part of PHE.

iii This was also phone calls – the analysis was just on phone calls to both systems (NHS111 took over the phone service part way through the analysis).
iv See Part 4.

References

1. Wikipedia. *Bills of Mortality*. Available at: https://en.wikipedia.org/wiki/Bills_of_mortality.
2. Wikipedia. *William Farr*. Available at: https://en.wikipedia.org/wiki/william_farr.
3. Wikipedia. *John Snow: Legacy and Honours*. Available at: https://en.wikipedia.org/wiki/John_Snow#Legacy_and_honours.
4. Wikipedia. *Florence Nightingale*. Available at: https://en.wikipedia.org/wiki/florence_nightingale.
5. GOV.UK. *Press Release: Sewage Signals Early Warning of Coronavirus Outbreaks*. Available at: www.gov.uk/government/news/sewage-signals-early-warning-of-coronavirus-outbreaks.
6. GOV.UK. *England Summary*. Available at: https://coronavirus.data.gov.uk/.
7. GOV.UK. Official Statistics: *Wider Impacts of COVID-19 on Health Monitoring Tool*. Available at: www.gov.uk/government/statistics/wider-impacts-of-covid-19-on-health-monitoring-tool.
8. NHS. *Get Running with Couch to 5k*. Available at: www.nhs.uk/live-well/exercise/running-and-aerobic-exercises/get-running-with-couch-to-5k/.
9. Office for Health Improvement & Disparities. *National General Practice Policies*. Available at: https://fingertips.phe.org.uk/profile/general-practice.
10. Marmot, M. *The Health Gap: The Challenges of an Unequal World*, Bloomsbury Publishing, 2016.
11. Wikipedia. *Local Area Agreement*. Available at: https://en.wikipedia.org.wiki/local_area_agreement.
12. Wikipedia. *National Support Teams*. Available at: https://en.wikipedia.org/wiki/National_Support_Teams.
13. GOV.UK. *The Public Health National Support Teams 2006–11*. Available at: www.gov.uk/government/publications/the-public-health-national-support-teams-2006-11.
14. Barr, B. Investigating the impact of the English health inequalities strategy: Time trend analysis, *BMJ*, 26 July 2017. Available at: https://doi.org/10.1136/bmj.j3310.
15. Abbas, J., Wrench, G. and Hennessey M. *From Data to Decisions: Building Blocks for Population Health Intelligence Systems*, 5 December 2018. Available at: https://ukhsa.blog.gov.uk/2018/12/05/from-data-to-decisions-building-blocks-for-population-health-intelligence-systems/.
16. The New York Times. *President Trump Is Unfit for This Crisis. Period*. Available at: https://nytimes.com/2020/03/09/opinion/trump-corona-cdc-html.
17. GOV.UK. *Data Job Family*. Available at: www.gov.uk/government/collections/digital-data-and-technology-profession-capability-framework#data-job-family.
18. NHS England. *Professionalisation*. Available at: https://transform.england.nhs.uk/key-tools-and-info/nhsx-analytics-unit/data-and-analytics-partnership-gateway/professionalisation/.

19. Glassdoor. *The UK's Top 15 Jobs with the Highest Satisfaction*. Available at: www.glassdoor.co.uk/blog/jobs-highest-satisfaction/.
20. Seed Scientific. How Much Data Is Created Every Day? +27 Staggering Stats. Available at: https://seedscientific.com/how-much-data-is-created-every-day/.
21. Faculty of Public Health. *National Public Health Specialty Training Recruitment*. Available at: www.fph.org.uk/training-careers/recruitment/recruitment-information/.

4 Healthcare public health

*Mahendra G. Patel; Yvonne Doyle; Anita Parkin;
Laura Bridle; Fiona Sim; Jenny Wright*

Introduction to this function

Healthcare public health (HCPH) professionals aim to improve and protect
patients' health and outcomes by reducing inequalities in the provision and
access to healthcare and in making sure that safe and effective services are
provided, and that the healthcare environment is one that promotes health
among patients, staff and visitors. Activities might include:

- developing specifications for services to be commissioned;
- advice on setting priorities for others to provide particular services;
- reviewing pathways to ensure services meet the needs of particular groups
  in the population;
- commissioning services;
- researching and advising on the evidence base for the effectiveness of services and particular treatments; and
- evaluating health outcomes of specific services.

The public health workforce in healthcare will work from a variety of settings, including the public sector – such as the NHS (hospital and community
providers, primary care, commissioning bodies and public health agencies),
local and central government, independent sector and academe. Increasingly,
the term 'population health management' is being used in the UK to describe
what has historically been part of the remit of HCPH, with a focus on using
information to support service redesign, in order better and more efficiently
to meet the needs of specific user groups.

Future challenges and opportunities – enhancing the role of healthcare public health

*Mahendra G. Patel, Professor and Pharmacy and Inclusion and
Diversity Lead, Department of Primary Care Health Sciences,
University of Oxford*

In my role as a pharmacist working in healthcare and in research, I have always aimed to impact public health through reducing health inequalities and

DOI: 10.4324/9781003433699-6

improving health outcomes, particularly for minority communities. Research and experience have both shown me that, to do this successfully, one must meaningfully and purposely reach out to the many underserved and disadvantaged groups in society that have been historically and incorrectly dubbed as so-called 'hard to reach'. Effective community engagement must be the message wherever we see inequalities, whether urban or rural. We need to understand, however, that communities differ not only in their needs, but also in the best way to engage with them and for them to subsequently effect positive change. This message has been further heightened recently through my work around the Coronavirus pandemic. This exposed early on that older people and people from ethnic minority origin were disproportionately adversely affected, while those with a learning disability were four times more likely than others to die from the virus.

During my career, I have worked extensively on diabetes and cardiovascular health with Black, Asian and Minority Ethnic (BAME) communities, developing toolkits, resources and literature in different languages, and working with the voluntary sector, including the British Heart Foundation (BHF) and the South Asian Health Foundation (SAHF). This experience proved invaluable during the pandemic, where it was quite clear that blanket messaging or, indeed, putting up a public health poster in a pharmacy, for example, did not always reach the diversity of communities that needed to hear the message – what to do, how to support one another, how to get tests and, then, when available, how to get the vaccine. Not everyone has a computer to get onto a government website or, as is the case with some in the Black and South Asian communities, has a great deal of trust in government messaging. I personally did regular media interviews to explain how to get tested, then vaccinated, on Pakistani radio and Punjabi TV stations to name but a few, where I became a trusted face, and for a number of Gujarati, Hindi, Urdu and Punjabi-speaking communities. Even if written messages are translated for different communities, not everyone is literate. What is needed, therefore, to protect people's health is a tailoring of messaging and also a tailoring of the means of messaging to suit different communities and cultures. This a complex area and we are not always culturally competent to appreciate how different communities live, their attitudes, behaviours, beliefs and understanding. A range of approaches, including using the power of different social media, is needed. Engaging with different faith groups can be a productive and more trusted way of conveying messages. I have also made use of university communities, especially those that are based in inner cities and areas of high deprivation. It's important we should always endeavour to work closely with national and local community and faith leaders wherever possible to help establish how best to reach their community and gain their trust; equally, with places of worship such as temples, gurdwaras, mosques, synagogues and churches. Notably, some faith communities were early adopters of the COVID-19 vaccine (for example, Hindus and Jews), and crucially, no major known religious authorities have banned vaccination.

During my work during 2020–2022 in raising awareness and aiding re-cruitment of volunteers from disadvantaged and diverse backgrounds for two major national trials testing new treatments for COVID-19,[1] commu-nity pharmacists proved invaluable 'foot-soldiers' in providing support and advice to many areas and communities that we often fail to reach out to. As well as supporting recruitment to research, community pharmacies and their teams have been critically important as a key local resource throughout the pandemic. On average, the majority of the population can access a local community pharmacy within a 20-minute walking distance. They are highly accessible and often open late at night and at weekends, with many being available on almost every high street in the country. Moreover, 44% of phar-macists and almost 14% of registered pharmacy technicians are themselves from ethnic minority backgrounds – they are better positioned to understand many of the different cultures and languages and can serve as a valuable interface. Pharmacists are a highly skilled and knowledgeable asset – not just in the community, but also in primary care and hospital settings when it comes to patient care, and understand closely the public health perspective. We should make better and further use, therefore, of their expertise and the wide-ranging pharmacy networks we have throughout the UK. With the sig-nificant changes in the NHS in 2022 and as we focus on providing a seamless and more accessible service for all patients wherever they live and whatever their background, the evolution of primary care networks (PCNs), and more recently the Integrated Care Systems (ICS) in England, have made it ex-tremely exciting for pharmacists to become more engaged with both clinical and preventive medicine.

Remember: one size does not fit all; one hit that works can be a very big hit!

Overview of the healthcare public health function

Yvonne Doyle, Medical Director for Public Health, NHS England

Why we need public health in the healthcare sector

It is very important to have public health in healthcare. Healthcare public health is, however, not a term widely understood and it is, perhaps, time to change this. What does matter is getting the health impact from healthcare and getting health service input into health. What can it do for the health of the population? We have to rethink not only the contemporary NHS, but any healthcare service. We must steer the thinking towards population health and what is appropriate in terms of preventive care as well as disease manage-ment. This, therefore, includes those who are not already patients, but who could become patients. There is currently a welcome push in the NHS to review its role in preventive care.

There are many different dimensions in addition to getting best outcomes for patients. The health service can contribute to population health as a major employer, for example. The health service should offer good 'people health' as part of the benefit of working in healthcare.

The public health role in preventive care

There is an offer every clinical person can make – a universal offer from the NHS of 'teachable moments' or 'making every contact count (MECC)' – which applies from A&E right through to preventive services in primary care. Clinicians take the opportunity during patient consultation to make people think about their own health and help prevent them from getting into trouble with their health later on. There are also preventive possibilities for people on waiting lists – 'stop before the op!' Clinicians can take the opportunity at every point to get people to pay more attention to their health. This could include, for example, smoking and pointing people to the well-evidenced pathway of tobacco cessation.

Public health professionals can help maximise this 'upstream' potential of the healthcare setting. This includes services such as screening and immunisation, as well as primary care in the community. Public health can also remind everyone working in or for the health service of the importance of tackling inequalities and disparities in health, as in the English policy called 'CORE20PLUS5'.[i]

Public health professionals can help get to the soul of every clinician by ensuring they ask who is benefitting from their service and are they doing the right thing by the right people? It is not just a case of responding to who shouts loudest, but about treating those with greatest needs – those who may have little voice.

What public health professionals can offer commissioning and providing healthcare

Qualified public health professionals have specialist knowledge to bring to bear on both commissioning and providing care to ensure the resulting services are equitable, of good quality, of maximum health benefit, effective and evidence-based. This runs from primary care through to specialist commissioning, where public health advice is highly valued, providing the evidence base for what is commissioned. The public health offer spans both commissioned and provided services. From a public health perspective, effective commissioning influences how care is identified and purchased, and which population it is provided to, and it also ensures clinicians offer preventive care. For provided care, they can ensure access is equitable and outcomes are measured and benefit the population.

Specialist services commissioning

There is a programme of commissioning spanning relatively rare to very rare services for which public health consultants lead the evidence-based commissioning. There are a few highly specialised public health posts at national level and some more at regional level. It is a very precious resource to spend on rarity. But it makes sure that there is a fair allocation of service. The evidence supporting decision making always has to be good enough to withstand potential legal challenge.

Population health management and public health

When I came back to work in the NHS in 2021, I found confusion over the terms 'population health management' as opposed to 'public health'. We need to explain the comprehensiveness of public health. Population health management refers largely to data and population segmentation for commissioning purposes. People can grasp that, but not the whole range of ways in which we use the data, how data turned into intelligence can make a difference to communities. That is what makes public health. Population health management is an important part of the public health function, just as prevention is, and refers to the industrialisation of data. Use of the term has, however, raised the game – the scale, the scope and the quality of data. This is not new: mapping infections was, after all, where public health started! Work on inequalities, prevention, public health commissioning, population health management and supporting clinicians and others to achieve high-quality outcomes together form a picture of what good healthcare public health looks like.

National work must dovetail with local systems

People must identify what they are adding at the level at which they are working. At the national level, it is connecting key programmes with a health benefit, convening diverse leaders towards collaboration, providing specialist advice and garnering evidence. Regions have a delivery arm in implementing big preventive healthcare programmes, as well as monitoring whether things are working well (or not), what is going on in the field and seeking how the national service can offer specialist help. Regional public health professionals share good practice across geographies – there is a lot of learning in place-based settings[ii] – doing it once for many. Part of my role now as NHS Medical Director for Public Health in England is to set up the appropriate networks for health to make sure all this is connected.

Much of public health work now resides in local government. We particularly need good connections between the NHS and local government at place level. In my role, I communicate regularly with colleagues in local government and the representative bodies for that sector. This is intended to be helpful, offering senior links in public health within the NHS, and reaching out to support good partnership work.

Healthcare public health professionals

There are some professionals who are dually qualified as clinicians and in public health. Public health professionals, typically, do not offer direct clinical care in their public health role, but can advise on the health impact of care.

It is valuable, but not essential, to have a clinical background before entering healthcare public health. Supporting MECC, for example, can be done from any background. Public health specialists who have a clinical background and can, therefore, more easily understand the context clinicians work in, may find it easier to gain credibility with clinical colleagues. It also helps, but again is not essential, if you can demonstrate that you are or have been active in research, if you can speak with authority to academics, particularly those working in teaching hospitals, on your particular understanding of what is good, and what is poor, quality evidence. Medicine can be hierarchical and you must show you can work with those who practise it at any level.

It is, therefore, important to keep your Continuing Professional Development (CPD) up to date so that you can talk to clinicians in their own language. For example, I am chair of the haematology board for one hospital trust. It is important the clinicians see me as an asset. What they want from public health is a balanced view. I am not one of them, but I also do not have a particular advocacy function. I know the evidence base, but understand the context clinicians are working in and I can provide an umbrella view of both commissioning and providing. I can help clinical colleagues find their way through the system. As Medical Director of a Strategic Health Authority for a number of years, I was involved in hospital restructuring, including mergers of specialist areas of work. Clinicians respected the fact that someone had to enable difficult decisions. It is the tricky end of the work. You have to be prepared for controversy and be quite brave, stating, for example, when changes may add little population benefit.

Healthcare public health can make a difference across the spectrum

Many Integrated Care Boards (ICBs) in England are looking for people with public health skills. Public health is not a statutory requirement on ICBs, but most Integrated Care Systems (the wider partnerships within which ICBs exist) are looking for public health skills at a senior level – not just for commissioning, but for the whole 'concept' of population health. We are, after all, building on the shoulders of giants. Regional directors of public health have been delivering for many years on tobacco, inequalities, obesity and violence reduction. Their team colleagues (deputy regional directors) are responsible for healthcare advice, have professional links to the screening services in regions and have oversight of quality assurance and measurement of outcomes.

We are now seeing falling life expectancy when in past decades we had been used to life expectancy continuing to rise, so what can healthcare public health do about it? We can work on cardiovascular programmes (prevention of heart disease and strokes), hypertension (high blood pressure) services and diabetes prevention programmes. These are major causes of premature mortality which impact unequally on the population of the UK. Public health can advise on the critical interventions we need to make before things deteriorate further, and ensure that population outcomes are kept in sight. A digital service for weight reduction has, for example, reached communities we did not think would be possible to reach, embracing all ages and backgrounds. Public health needs, then, to ensure the delivery chains are secured, providing a sound pathway and effective, timely referral.

Local Falls Prevention Services, recommending physical activity to prevent muscle deterioration and to offset frailty in care homes, are run jointly between public health and clinicians. Preventing falls can offset hospital admissions, which is important for the NHS, as well as patients.

There is also a strong link to health protection. When I was leading the health protection service in Public Health England (PHE), for example, there was a listeria food poisoning outbreak linked to hospital food. This led to a national programme to improve the quality of all hospital food. Better nutrition helps people get out of hospital faster. In my current role, I have reached out to the UK Heath Security Agency (UKHSA) and Directors of Public Health (DsPH) from local government to solve how we develop a more coherent approach to health protection within the NHS and between it and other parts of the health system, so that we can deliver joined-up pathways, where roles and responsibilities are clearer.

Getting into healthcare public health

It helps if you like the setting and enjoy working with colleagues from a wide range of disciplines caring for patients as they get through the system. But you need to be able to look beyond that – to be entrepreneurial, to have a focus on equity, to be the conscience of the NHS and to ask the 'so what' questions – to understand the impact of services on health. It is also helpful to learn about and experience frontline services in some part of your higher professional training.

Those working in healthcare public health are relatively small in number and you have to work through others – to explain the value of health as an asset to society and what the setting can do to help each individual's own health. There is a scientific and a service element. It is importantly also about relationship building and partnership working with the NHS and between the NHS and its essential partners – for example, local government, Royal Colleges, the National Institute for Health and Care Excellent (NICE) and UKHSA.

It is exciting and an opportunity to be influential in the healthcare setting. People working in healthcare public health are 'in it and of it' and can give a steer which can benefit the public's health. It is much more difficult to do this from the outside.

My advice to the next generation

Stick with public health as a function. I didn't know what it was when I was a clinician, but I felt there was something interesting and exciting beyond clinical work. If you are interested in the health of the population – come to us, join us and then stay with us! A career in public health will endlessly sustain your curiosity.

Personal reflections

It is a privilege to have held the roles I have had from being a consultant through to national leadership work as Medical Director and Director of Health Protection for Public Health England during the pandemic, and now as a public health leader in the NHS. The pandemic was hard, but there was nowhere I would rather have been, in there doing my bit.

My career path

When I qualified as a doctor in Dublin in 1981, I felt the natural environment was poorly looked after – buses spewing out a lot of rubbish while I was riding behind them on my bike. As a junior surgeon in a rural hospital, I came across numbers of people being admitted in the summer following severe farm accidents. I started collecting information on this and eventually my research got published. This led to some awards. I still didn't know much about public health until someone said I should do it – to get paid to do this kind of work all the time! So I trained in public health in Dublin, then moved with my family to London when I got a research job in 1989.

From there, I did numerous jobs in the NHS, Department of Health and Social Care (DHSC), academia and the independent sector. I was a Director of Public Health (DPH) at one point, covering three boroughs in South West London, a job I loved. It was place-based and made me very aware of the breadth of the public health service offer, including health protection.

Between 2013 and 2019, I was Statutory Advisor to two Mayors of London and, from 2019, Medical Director and Director of Health Protection for PHE, leading the English public health service through the pandemic. Currently, I am NHS Medical Director for Public Health, leading the public health national function within the NHS in England. As a senior public health doctor in NHS England, I provide leadership for professional standards and public health services throughout the NHS.

I have a particular research and policy interest in sustainable global cities and in mortality, life expectancy and international analyses of the COVID-19 pandemic.

Career stories

Anita Parkin, Director of Population Health, Central London Community Healthcare NHS Trust

There is, currently (February 2023), no statutory requirement for a public health function in the provider sector in the NHS, but many trusts have a public health function of some type.

I began my public health career as a public health analyst and progressed through various analytical roles subsequently, qualifying as a public health consultant via the portfolio route as one of the very early specialist registrars on the UK Public Health Registrants (UKPHR) register. I came into public health via my passion to work in the NHS, using my skills, qualifications and experience in statistics and health economics, and developed specialism in the analysis of health inequalities during the 1990s.

I have held a variety of posts in various English NHS regions, working in epidemiological roles. I also held three very different DPH roles over 20 years as a joint director of public health in the NHS and local government and latterly as a local government director of public health.

As I now move towards the end of a long public health career, I have stepped into an NHS provider public health role, which has brought interesting and unexpected challenges, enriched in a perverse way by the COVID-19 pandemic.

My own role in moving to a very large provider trust following many years as a conventional DPH was initially to bring some of the more general population health skills and analytical insights to a huge staff cohort working in frontline roles, many of which are essentially community public health roles, such as health visitors, school nurses and district nurses.

My transition into the NHS coincided exactly with the COVID-19 pandemic, which inevitably entailed the use of my infection control and epidemiological skills and experience in outbreak management. Like many other public health colleagues, this was a gruelling challenge, but it produced an incredible opportunity to engage with the trust staff from the frontline to the executive and the non-executives.

As the trust has emerged from the pandemic, while some things may never quite be the same post COVID-19, there is a legacy of public health engagement and a place for public health that has been firmly established. I have established, for example, an online staff population health training course and a public health analytical function, and my own role stretches across the many facets of health inequalities and clinical outcomes.

I continue to be registered as a public health consultant and the transferable knowledge gained in my many years working as an NHS public health consultant and a local government public health consultant has made the transition, and the opportunity to engage with partners and on partnership projects, invaluable. NHS trusts inevitably cover different boundaries and overlapping areas of geography and responsibility, and this diversity adds to the richness of undertaking this type of role.

While my last 30 years in public health have been busy as well as challenging, they have been rewarding and I have no regrets about the career path I have taken. It has been influenced by legislative and organisational and structural changes that have shaped how public health is delivered. It has also been influenced by epidemiological changes, good, bad and unpredictable-but-not-unexpected events such as swine flu and COVID-19, as well as general changes and preventive healthcare. While I had an outline plan for a public health career, flexibility – both personal and career wise – and to some extent physical mobility, that is a willingness to move to new roles, have enabled to me to achieve some level of work/life balance and satisfaction on both fronts. This has also been helped by the most recent changes, the acceleration of the use of IT and remote technology, enabling distant working across large organisations and collaboration with partners.

Laura Bridle, Public Health Consultant Midwife

How I started in public health

My passion for public and population health started when I began my training as a nurse in Canada in 2003. I had the privilege of working across different areas and disciplines and loved the impact you could see when services came together. Once qualified, I worked for Toronto Public Health as a nurse and had two projects working with the homeless population and running a tuberculosis surveillance service for newly arrived migrants. Being able to visit the shelters brought it home very quickly why many had chosen the streets over the apparent safety of a shelter. There was risk of violence, theft and drug use, and an increased risk of catching tuberculosis (TB). This made health so complex, that we could screen and educate around TB, but if you did not have the support of social services and the funding bodies, there was little benefit. I later worked as an obstetric nurse on a postnatal ward. Pregnancy and birth are such crucial times to make a positive impact on someone's experience of healthcare and health promotion. You are not just supporting the woman and family – but you are also helping support the environment this new life would be coming into. This is where I first met a midwife – a very new profession in Canada, with the first midwife registered in 1994 – and made the decision to return to the UK to train and work as a midwife.

Once qualified, I started work as a caseload midwife in London, UK and got to support women and birthing people from their first pregnancy booking appointment up until 28 days post-birth. I could see the impact midwives could offer women and families, as we help to ensure a healthy pregnancy and good start for their newborn. I also recognised the impact social determinants played on pregnancy. These include ethnicity, age, income, education, pre-pregnancy health and housing. While spending seven months working with Médecins Sans Frontières (MSF) in South Sudan, I witnessed the impact of war and displacement, but most importantly the importance of working with communities to ensure health education can be shared and that services can be shaped to meet the needs and expectations of those we support.

Moving into public health research as a midwife

When I returned again to London, I started an MSc in advanced practice midwifery and this opened not only my mind, but also doors to meeting other colleagues whom I continue to look up to today. I completed modules in international women's mental health, leadership and research. This enabled me to conduct my own qualitative research and publish work that has meant ongoing development and change in the care we give women in the UK with little to no English. I completed a Post Graduate Certificate in Perinatal Mental Health and was later accepted into Health Education England (HEE)'s population health fellowship for one year.[2] This fellowship was a wonderful opportunity and I am continuing to work with colleagues on projects that were co-created from my time in South East (SE) London. This was my first introduction to population health management and the impact having access to near real-time data can achieve.

One of my projects was looking to improve the uptake of postnatal surveillance of type II diabetes in women with a history of gestational diabetes. Women with this history have a 50% chance of developing type II diabetes within the first five years post-birth.[3] After speaking to women, it became evident that despite Black and Asian women being at increased risk of both gestational and type II diabetes, the information being shared with them was not culturally sensitive and the importance of post-natal screening was not being made clear.[4] The NHS Long Term Plan (2019) set out new commitments to strengthen the role of the NHS in the prevention of ill health and reduction of health inequalities.[5] For example, women were being given the diagnosis in pregnancy, but being given White European recipes to use, and for the population in SE London, this was not appropriate or effective. One woman said to me: 'What am I supposed to do? I work part-time and have to cook for my kids, I am not going to make two or three different meals.' Working with GPs, diabetic nurses, dieticians, medical consultants and, most importantly, women and birthing people, we have co-created a culturally sensitive recipe book that has been funded to ensure those accessing maternity care in SE London can be offered a free hard or digital copy of the book. Due to the success of the book, we have also been granted permission, by the SE London Clinical Commissioning Group (CCG) who funded the project, to share the resource nationally.[6]

My second project was related to medication for mental illness in pregnancy. Anecdotally, I was seeing women and birthing people become unwell after abruptly stopping their usual medication or not being prescribed any after their GP had told them it was not safe in pregnancy. I used population health management to discover that almost two-thirds of women (n=174) stopped their psychotropic medication within the first three months of pregnancy over a one-year period in one SE London borough. I created a multidisciplinary working group, including a GP, pharmacist, psychiatrist, health visitor and, most importantly again, the voices of women and birthing people through the local maternity 'voice partnership'. We ran a GP-led survey in 2020 which confirmed that not all GPs are confident to prescribe antidepressants in pregnancy. Furthermore, it appeared that many GPs were not aware of the specialist services or help available. As part of the survey, GPs were asked if access to a decision aid would help increase their confidence to prescribe antidepressants in pregnancy. The response was 'yes'. We then came together to co-create two resources produced by our expert stakeholder group:

1 a poster for women informing them to not stop this medication without discussion; and
2 an information guide for GPs, including links to how to refer and/or get advice about prescribing from their local dedicated perinatal pharmacist helpline.

The information for women about this is available to them via their midwife and includes relevant hyperlinks to resources such as BUMPS and Tommy's charity.[7] The poster and design was funded and is showcased in pharmacies, maternity wards, GP practices and sexual health clinics in SE London. NHS Communication Teams have been consulted and agreed to the final design of the poster. This needed to go through consultation with mental health services in SE London prior to the official launch. The process was long, but we are delighted to have this freely available not just for SE London, but also nationally, with the understanding that contact information of perinatal mental health teams will need to be edited to match the location of the service using it.

More recent public health roles

Since the fellowship in 2020/21, I finished a six-month secondment as a public health consultant midwife, where I was able to introduce training on improving the care we give to Black women in pregnancy and beyond, through support from the Five X More campaign. MBRRACE-UK is a national audit programme and is commissioned by all four UK governments to collect information about all late foetal losses, stillbirths, neonatal deaths and maternal deaths across the UK.[iii] The report has highlighted decades of inequity in outcomes for Black, Asian and mixed-race women and babies, Black women currently being four times more likely to die in childbirth. This is why this training is so very important, so we can look at ways we can change this narrative. The report has highlighted further risk for those who need to access language support services. I helped support the development of training around the use of interpreter services as a Special Clinical Advisor for the Maternity Clinical Network in London, which has been offered nationally and completed in early 2023. I currently work as a senior midwife within the maternal mental health service, where I am supporting five hospitals in SE London leading on care pathways and improving service provision.

Advice to the next generation

1 Writing and publishing is very important to showcase the work you do in public and population health, not only for your own career progression, but also to allow for others hoping or already doing similar work to share ideas. Due to my experience and work, I have contributed to a book

around migrant health which was published in 2022. I have published three articles from work surrounding my fellowship. I published articles from both my BSc and MSc dissertations. I recommend that you write and bring colleagues in to help you. Publications are also important if you want a future career as a consultant midwife, for example, or to gain access to fellowships or academic roles.

2 Apply for funding. It is expensive to attend conferences and undertake further education,[iv] but they are both great ways to learn about exciting new projects, as well as meet colleagues from across the UK, if not further afield. See Useful Resources for information about where you can get access to grants, but do speak to your local Trust or university as well. I was fortunate to get my MSc dissertation module funded by Nightingale Fund and attend the International Conference of Midwives Triennial Congress thanks to Iolanthe Midwifery Trust.

And the future?

My ambition for the future is to complete my PhD and work the remainder of my days as a clinical academic. I love being in the community and working clinically, but I also really enjoy being part of making sustainable change and improvements in care. This career path allows for both. I would recommend any midwife interested in a career in public or population health to say 'yes'. If there are opportunities to be involved in a research project, present at a conference, or apply for a fellowship or additional education, do it. Do not be afraid. So many of us have, and I continue to have, imposter syndrome. For this very reason, I would also encourage that if you are able to access opportunities you bring others up with you. The work and ideas that come from a diverse workforce are endless.

Notes

i An NHS England approach to reducing health inequalities at both national and local system level which defines a target population cohort from the most deprived 20% of the national population, plus specific population groups such ethnic minorities and inclusion health groups, and identifies '5' focus clinical areas requiring accelerated improvement.
ii Place-based approaches look at the characteristics of local places as the starting point for planning and the communities within each place, focusing efforts collaboratively to make the biggest impact.
iii MBRRACE-UK: Mothers and Babies: Reducing risk through audits and confidential enquiries across the UK https://www.npeu.ox.ac.uk/mbrrace-uk
iv See Chapter 14.

References

1. PRINCIPLE (March 2020) and PANORAMIC (December 2021), UK-wide clinical studies sponsored by the University of Oxford and funded by the National

Institute for Health Research to find effective COVID-19 treatments. Available at: www.principletrial.org and www.panoramictrial.org respectively.

2. NHS Health Education England. *Population Health Fellowship*. Available at: www.hee.nhs.uk/our-work/population-health/population-health-fellowship-0.

3. NICE. *Diabetes in Pregnancy: Management from Preconception to the Postnatal Period*, 2015. Available at: www.nice.org.uk/guidance/ng3.

4. Herrick, C.J., Puri, R., Rahaman, R., Hardi, A., Stewart, K. and Colditz, G.A. Maternal race/ethnicity and postpartum diabetes screening: A systematic review and meta-analysis. *J. Women's Health* (Larchmt), 2020; 29(5): 609–21.

5. NHS. *NHS Long Term Plan*. Available at: www.longtermplan.nhs.uk.

6. NHS South East London. *Culturally Sensitive Cookbook for Women and Birthing People with Gestational Diabetes*. Available at: https://selondonccg.nhs.uk/news/culturally-sensitive-cookbook-for-women-and-birthing-people-with-gestational-diabetes-free/.

7. Best use of Medicine in Pregnancy (BUMPS). Available at: https://medicinesinpregnancy.org/. See also Tommy's. Available at: www.tommys.org/.

5 Health protection

Tracy Daszkiewicz; Andrew Jones; Giri Shankar;
David Roberts; Oluwakemi Olufon; Fiona Sim;
Jenny Wright

Introduction to this function

Health protection specialists and practitioners protect the safety of the whole
population. This can include:

- protecting people from infectious diseases;
- food safety;
- protecting people from environmental hazards, such as noise, air and water pollution, biological, chemical or radiation;
- safety in the workplace; and
- emergency preparedness and response.

During the COVID-19 pandemic, the crucial role of protecting people from
infectious disease came to the fore, with specialists and practitioners providing
professional leadership and advice to hospitals, GPs, councils and the greater
NHS, care homes and members of the public, and contacting those most at risk.
Infectious disease epidemiologists played a key public-facing role in monitoring
the course of the pandemic and modelling potential future paths of the virus.

The health protection public health workforce is principally located within
the NHS, local government and civil service, depending on the different con-
figurations in each UK country. In each, the frontline workforce is backed by
laboratory scientists. The UK Health Security Agency (UKHSA), an executive agency of the Department of Health and Social Care (DHSC) for public
health protection and infectious disease capability in England, has a UK-wide
coordinating role with Public Health Scotland, Public Health Wales and the
Northern Ireland Public Health Agency.

Future challenges and opportunities – vision for the health protection function

Tracy Daszkiewicz, Executive Director of Public Health, Aneurin
Bevan University Hospital Board, Gwent, Wales

The greatest challenge facing the public health workforce now is capacity
and securing a workforce for the future. All the work public health has

DOI: 10.4324/9781003433699-7

done, and led, during the pandemic has not resulted in sustainable public health provision. In England, we have breadth in that the workforce is located in so many different organisations – within the DHSC, the UK UKHSA and the Office for Health Improvement & Disparities (OHID), and in local government and the NHS. This breadth can be used to enhance interdisciplinary working across the domains of public health. It could also be seen as a weakness – in that the workforce is so fragmented. The previous structure, Public Health England (PHE), set up at the time of the Health and Social Care Act (2012), was developed as a national body to pull the domains together. Time will tell if elements have been lost and what has been gained. It seems clear, though, that the UKHSA will not have the same funding going forward as it had during the pandemic. This is likely to create a challenge for horizon-scanning for future risks and having the capacity in place to deal with effective mitigation, response and recovery of future pandemics. What we do know from the 2012 reorganisation, however, is that the strength of public health is in making things work. Many of us were nervous, for example, about moving from the NHS into local government in 2013, but we have seen the benefits of working across an integrated agenda and being part of local government has brought a great deal of benefit. Our priority now is to ensure public health is well positioned to support the health agenda through having a strong voice with the new NHS Integrated Care Systems (ICS) in England from July 2022 and, especially in the absence of a statutory public health position at ICS Board level, to ensure standardised engagement of public health and to be part of this structure as a partner of equals.

I was a Director of Public Health (DPH) in local government when the pandemic started. The first couple of months were mainly focused on establishing monitoring systems to alert Elected Members of any cases. By March, structures were put in place and DsPH chaired the Strategic Co-ordinating Group to set up the local response structures. The leadership for response was very local in the early months, with local government putting services in place to meet the needs of their populations, based very much on place-based values. I had secured a new role with PHE which I delayed by a couple of months, leaving in June 2020 to take up a role leading population health with a focus on health inequalities and recovery. A significant amount of the role was surge capacity for health protection and working with them to streamline calls and queries. I benefitted from seeing the pandemic response through these different lenses and the public health family working together at all levels. I moved back to local government in December 2021, having missed having a direct line to the community.

In health protection, it is the magic of the people we work with which makes all the difference. Those who specialise in health protection are phenomenal technicians with skill and expertise. I have worked alongside the best. When the surge came during the pandemic, those working in local government and regional public health teams on other programmes such as health improvement moved to work on health protection to increase capacity and give the technical experts space to focus on the more complex situations. This helped identify those socially isolated, including those who had mental health or financial issues. The disciplines all gelled and became interdependent. Everyone's expertise was needed. People for whom health protection was not their first discipline learned quickly to answer the extraordinary volume and complexity of questions from the public on the phone, gave information, provided briefings for schools and undertook thematic analysis. Practitioners and also those in administration were all involved. As we move beyond the pandemic I hope these skills can be maintained through continuing professional development (CPD).[i]

Previously, as DPH, I had seen this readiness of public health and others to respond during the nerve agent poisonings in Salisbury in 2018. I was part of a well-established Local Resilience Forum and we had strength from our training and exercises in emergency response. We knew where the expertise was and when the call came we rallied. We had the right skill mix and the right mix of personalities leading the different strategic and operational groups involved. I worked closely with PHE, co-chairing the scientific and technical advisory group. The strategic and technical group chairs remained the same during the incidents, while organisations refreshed the staff involved by rotating them through different roles. The partnership working was phenomenal. Individual expertise was always at the table, but no decision was made unilaterally, we worked through the evidence and all brought our specialisms around the collective aim of protecting our community. As DPH, I take my role of protecting the health of the population very seriously. I learned a lot from this incident; as in other major events I had worked on, the defining aspect was the number of those injured or killed. We did not have many casualties fortunately and one fatality, but I learned that one is too big a number. This is the hardest aspect of having worked on this incident. I still struggle with it. We keep going because it is our job, but it can be hard.

I have reflected a lot on how we worked during 2018, while all professions and roles have pulled together and worked differently to meet the demands of a new way of working and living. People have been and are working incredibly hard and we need to look after the emotional health of all those who have had to work throughout and deal with anxiety, missing loved ones, those such as supermarket workers, postal officials and many more who have not been furloughed, but have kept us fed and connected, and, in the case of healthcare colleagues, greater exposure to illness and death. As someone who was 'spent' for a while myself after Salisbury, I can recognise that people working in health and social care are exhausted after two years of pandemic and need time to recover and reflect. We must not forget that returning to 'business as usual' depends on the very same people who are exhausted right now (in 2022) and need space for their own recovery!

I was impressed how our public health teams could move in and out of role, be flexible and step into the space that needed to be filled and work the hours required and just keep going. It is a multidisciplinary workforce with multiple layers and we do not normally work to a 'command and control' model; instead, we step into the spaces where we add the most value and pull together.

Now, we need to develop the workforce to increase capacity. There are currently two routes to specialist status – the portfolio and the training routes.[ii] Public health leaders, including DsPH in local authorities, need to be spotting talent and targeting people in their teams to be nominated for the practitioners' programme with mentor support from within the team. And we should encourage those working at higher grades who have a great deal of work experience and an appropriate background, but who are not aiming for the training scheme, to follow the portfolio route. We need to build the support into teams to help people do this, as for most they will be building their portfolio alongside a full-time role. All these avenues will help secure the capacity in the system for the future. Another way to increase capacity in local government is to grow public health skills among those working in other departments, such as planning, housing and safe-guarding.

I started out in social care, specialising in HIV, then working with young people and schools, challenging stigma and myths. This led to preventive work with children with complex needs, particularly those at risk of being drawn into criminal behaviour and sexual exploitation, and in alternative education settings. I was frustrated there were not the policies to support them and moved into roles where I thought I would be able to influence decision making. That is when I moved into public health roles, first as a sexual health strategist working in a Primary Care Trust (PCT), then working as Local Strategic Partnership Manager to look across at the environment, economy, built environment, health and education. It was from here I joined the Wiltshire Public Health team and I was sponsored to complete a Master's degree in Public Health (MPH) (thanks to my then DPH!). I was subsequently able to qualify for accreditation as a Defined Specialist on the UK Public Health Register after completing a retrospective portfolio of my work. I submitted my portfolio in 2014 and had an Acting Consultant in Public Health role while my portfolio was being assessed. In May the following year, I took up the Acting DPH role, securing the role substantively in December 2017.

My message: public health is an incredible profession with incredible people in it. Every day is different, and we work with amazing partners to improve and protect the health of our communities. No two days are the same, and to borrow the mantra from the Wiltshire Local Resilience Forum: 'We do the unusual in the usual way.'

Overview of the health protection function

Andrew Jones, Deputy National Director of Health Protection and Screening Services, Public Health Wales and Giri Shankar, Director of Health Protection, Public Health Wales

What is the health protection function?

Health protection is described (in the UK) as one of the three domains of public health practice and is recognised by the World Health Organization (WHO) as one of the ten essential public health operations.

Health protection is also a core function of global health security, coordinated through the International Health Regulations (IHR) 2005, to provide an overarching legal framework for handling public health events and emergencies that have the potential to cross borders. Following the departure of the UK from the European Union (EU), health security and health protection functions have been included in a Trade and Cooperation Agreement with the development of a Common Framework Policy and new UK legislation designed to address cross-border threats to health.

The health protection function involves actions for clean air, water and food, infectious disease control, protection against environmental health hazards, chemical incidents and emergency response. These activities include: *proactive* prevention functions (for example, infectious disease outbreak prevention and control, emergency planning); *reactive* acute response functions (risk management, communication of threats to health, infection management, outbreak and incident response); and some functions that span both (such as immunisation). Health protection is underpinned by 'information for action', with communicable disease and environmental surveillance functions established at country and international levels which serve as early warning and programme monitoring systems.[iii] The COVID-19 pandemic, and potential threats from biological, chemical and radiation agents including risks associated with conflict, demonstrate the importance of effective national and local health protection surveillance and response functions.

In the UK, health protection practice requires strong collaborative working between all levels (national, regional and local) and between agencies, including the NHS, local authorities, the voluntary sector and other partners, including Animal Health, the Food Standards Agency and the Health and Safety Executive.

Leading the above requires adaptable specialist knowledge and skills able to react to new emerging threats and technological advances. An effective health protection service therefore demands a 'fit for purpose' workforce educated and trained to the highest standards.

The contribution made to public health by health protection

The organisation and delivery of health protection functions has evolved over time in response to a changing burden of disease, population needs, emerging evidence and government policies. Broadly, health protection services cover the following areas:

- provision of specialist advice in the management of cases, incidents and outbreaks of notifiable infections and non-infectious environmental hazards, including rapid risk assessments and operational responses;
- undertaking high-quality surveillance and field epidemiology to generate 'information for action';
- teaching, training, research and development; and
- proactive partnership working on issues that impact on society's ability to protect its population's health, ranging from improving vaccination uptake, sexual health, health and justice, reducing antimicrobial resistance, emergency preparedness and health inequalities.

While we have tackled some of the biggest infectious disease threats in humankind's history, including polio and smallpox, the COVID-19 pandemic reminds us that the detection and control of infectious diseases is an ongoing and evolving story, including the rapid increases in the rate of drug (antibiotic) resistance in numerous infectious pathogens.

In our globalised world, where physical interactions between people are faster and more common than ever before, infectious diseases can spread far and wide in a short space of time. Running parallel to these challenges is the development of new technologies that will bring marked enhancements to our detection and control capabilities. These include rapid communications and whole genome sequencing, which provide us with the tools to share information and advice rapidly, bringing greater accuracy to our investigations.

The untapped potential to transform the way in which health protection services of the twenty-first century can be delivered is therefore enormous. This requires strengthened education and workforce development strategies to develop a dynamic, flexible and multi-disciplinary workforce that is both responsive to local needs and is able to make maximum use of digital technology (for example, artificial intelligence, mobile-phone-based monitoring of treatments), big data (for example, for targeted vaccinations) and empowered information (for example, user-defined shareable information).

Roles and career opportunities

As in other aspects of public health, there is a diverse range of roles within health protection, with the potential for career progression from entry level to senior leadership. For the purpose of illustration: a health protection team is a multi-disciplinary team comprising roles including: specialists/consultants; health protection nurses and practitioners; surveillance, field epidemiology and analytical staff; scientists; and trainees and, more recently (in England), apprentices, who, typically, work closely with partners, including environmental health practitioners, hospital microbiologists, infection control nurses, GPs and academic institutions.

Teams address all types of health hazards, but key areas of expertise include: immunisation; food- and water-borne diseases; respiratory infections; environmental hazards; and healthcare-acquired infections, with the provision of 24/7 emergency advice to healthcare professionals.

Going forward, roles and responsibilities within health protection teams will continue to experience major changes with new opportunities and skill mix. This is already being factored into national frameworks for education and development, such as in Scotland.

Health protection consultants are registered public health specialists.[iv] Health protection practitioners form part of the wider public health practitioner workforce. There are no set entry requirements or specific training routes to become a public health practitioner. The Faculty of Public Health (FPH) describes an example entry route as requiring 'a qualification and experience working in a public health-related area'.[1] For health protection, this could include a first level degree in public health, nursing or environmental health, or working in a knowledge and intelligence role. For more senior practitioner posts, a Master's Degree and registration with the UK Public Health Register (UKPHR) is often a requirement.[v] There are approved standards for practice, including specific standards for health protection (see Function A3 of the Public Health Skills and Knowledge Framework (PHSKF),[2] and there are examples of accredited training programmes supporting these.

The NHS Careers website provides a useful insight into other career roles in public health and many of these are nursing careers, including health protection nurses. The Royal College of Nursing (RCN) has developed useful resources on becoming a nurse and specifically on careers in public health nursing. A useful resource has been developed by NHS Scotland specifically for career development in health protection nursing.

The value of Environmental Health Practitioners as a critical part of the health protection workforce has been highlighted by the COVID-19 pandemic response. This is an exciting and dynamic career. A guide to accessing a career in environmental health is provided by the Chartered Institute of Environmental Health and includes advice in relation to study at school, college, university degree and apprenticeships, with excellent employment potential.

In recent years, apprenticeships in general public health (including for health protection practitioner roles) have also become available in England. These salaried posts (usually 36 months) facilitate integrated degree-level education and vocational training and lead to practitioner registration with UKPHR.[vi] Public health apprenticeship opportunities are also being developed in Wales.

Scientists, including data analysts, form a vital part of the health protection team. There is a comprehensive framework, Modernising Scientific Careers (MSC, last updated in 2022),[3] which outlines a UK-wide education and training strategy for the whole healthcare science workforce in the NHS and associated bodies. MSC introduces a clear and coherent career pathway and structure for the healthcare science workforce. Aspects of the programme cover every step of the career pathway, and include education, training and workforce planning.

We have described above some of the specialist roles in the health protection workforce. In doing so, we also respect the contribution of the local public health department to protecting the public's health. The COVID-19 pandemic has highlighted the need to ensure that this workforce can be rapidly and appropriately upskilled to provide surge response during national health protection emergencies.

Health protection achievements

In the UK, each of the four national governments has a Chief Medical Officer (CMO), whose key responsibility is to act as an advocate for population health and advise their respective ministers on policy matters. At regional and local level, Directors of Public Health have a key role in working with partners and local politicians to shape everyday policy and resource decisions to protect the health of the populations they serve.

There are several notable achievements within the UK and worldwide where public health specialists have made a tangible difference to protecting the health of the population.

Most recently, the COVID-19 pandemic has highlighted the critical role of the health protection, environmental health and general public health workforce in the UK response.

Other achievements include the contributions to polio eradication, and control of tropical diseases such as Malaria, Ebola and MERS-CoV. The rapid development of viral vector and mRNA vaccines for COVID-19 and delivery through mass population vaccination programmes have been lifesaving.

Environmental Health Protection has become recognised as a specialty within broader public health and has contributed to significant population-level interventions to tackle issues such as food safety, air pollution, safe housing and sustainability. The COVID-19 pandemic has similarly highlighted the need for a comprehensive and integrated focus on human, animal and environmental health ('One Health')[4] for the future.

My career journey – Andrew Jones

My personal career story spans all domains of public health, but starts with and is currently in health protection. This demonstrates the variety of opportunities available in this exciting career pathway, which has enabled me to live my values, working locally, regionally and nationally, for both local government and the NHS. I have constantly acquired additional knowledge/skills and undertaken technical, educational and leadership roles within a Wales/UK-wide multi-agency system. Each career stage has provided a rewarding job role and opportunities to undertake CPD. Working as a Local Authority Environmental Health Practitioner enabled me to make a difference to local communities, working on a diverse range of public protection issues, including food safety, housing and environmental control. My role as a 'meat hygiene inspector', for example, developed my key understanding of 'One Health', with the essential links between humans, animals and our environment.

A Master's degree in Public Health sparked my passion for epidemiology and ambition to become part of a multi-professional public health leadership workforce. As the first registered specialist (UKPHR portfolio route) from a background other than medicine, I have been rewarded with a mixed technical and leadership portfolio. Specialising first as a Consultant in Environmental Public Health, I developed to become an Executive Director of Public Health, where my wider strategic remit enabled me to advocate for the health of the population, influencing service development and resource allocation to tackle health inequalities. Specialising again as a Director of Health Protection and Microbiology, I have been privileged to work alongside multidisciplinary and clinical teams, collaborating with local authority partners, most recently in a truly testing pandemic response.

My current role as a Deputy National Director of Health Protection and Screening Services for Public Health Wales provides opportunities for system leadership at national, UK and international level, including working with the Chief Medical Officer and peers across the four nations of the UK. In my other role, as the current chair of UKPHR, I am committed to developing the standards for and regulation of our profession. After nearly 40 years of learning and practice, I remain passionate about this career and am focused on helping to develop a resilient health protection workforce for the twenty-first century.

My career journey – Giri Shankar

My passion for public health was ignited in my third year of medical school, when I was involved in India's polio eradication programme. The ability to achieve population-level health improvement, as distinct from individual patient level, is fascinating. That lay the foundations for choosing a career in public health. Over the past 22 years, I have had the opportunity to work in India, the UK (both England and Wales) and Europe. This rich experience has led to a much deeper understanding of population-level interventions, especially around vaccine-preventable diseases, field epidemiology, outbreak response and surveillance, which are cornerstones of health protection practice. Added to this is the ability to undertake operational research to answer grass-roots-level questions. The most satisfying part of the career for me is the ability to undertake 'detective' type work to solve disease outbreaks and the ability to influence health inequalities in a positive way through vaccination.

The practice of public health/health protection varies across different countries and continents. An inseparable part of public health practice is the link to politics and public policy. These are often dictated by resource allocation. My reflection of working in resource-scarce settings is that it leads to innovative practices, and focuses less on paperwork and documentation, but more on outcomes. In resource-rich settings, things can be relatively better organised, there can be more emphasis on clinical governance, record keeping, communication, training and reflection. During the immediate past couple of years, in fulfilling the role of an Incident Director for the COVID-19 response, I was able to experience, first-hand, a positive working relationship with the Chief Medical Officer (CMO) for Wales, the Chief Scientific Officer (CSO) for health and several other partners. The ability to use scientific evidence to influence public policy was immensely gratifying. Added to this, as a nominated public spokesperson for my organisation, the importance of communicating scientific messages in an easy-to-understand manner to our communities was challenging, but very rewarding, professionally.

Career stories

David Roberts, Consultant in Health Protection, UKHSA

(Please note: the views and opinions below are those of Dr Roberts, and do not necessarily represent the views or position of the UKHSA.)

How I started my career in public health

I officially started my public health career when I began the Public Health Specialty Training programme in Thames Valley in 2013. A medic by background, I had been interested in a public health career since medical school at the University of Birmingham, where I had excelled in the related disciplines of epidemiology and statistics, and in my fifth year I had completed a special study module with the public health team in my local Heart of Birmingham Primary Care Trust (where local public health teams were based at the time).

At that point, the experience confirmed that although there was plenty to interest me in the specialty, I wasn't ready to commit to leaving faster-paced patient-facing work until later on in my medical career. It was not until about six years into postgraduate medicine that I was ready to apply for public health training. By then, I was working as a clinical research fellow in immunology and infection in Cardiff on a clinical trial, as well as being on the general medical registrar hospital on-call rota.

The trials work gave me an opportunity to step away from the clinical environment into research, develop skills in epidemiology and statistics, and think about my career options. At the same time, I was becoming more conscious of health inequality and felt there was relatively little I could do in clinical medicine, but wondered if it was more of a focus within public health. I decided to do a taster week with the local health protection team, who very kindly let me shadow their work, which was primarily in communicable disease control, as well as introducing me to current registrars. They told me about their training, which sounded fantastic and included a funded

Master's course and placements working on all sorts of public health issues, ranging from the local level, but also to national health topics. It sounded perfect for my interests in infectious diseases, health inequalities, and aptitude in epidemiology and statistics, and I applied successfully to gain a place on the Thames Valley scheme, where my wife and I planned to move to live closer to family.

My early experience/relevant courses and qualifications obtained

I came into public health as a qualified medical doctor and with Membership of the Royal College of Physicians, as well as an interest in evidence-based medicine and clinical epidemiology, all of which stood me in good stead for the initial application and beyond. Almost immediately on starting public health training, registrars who have not already completed a Master's in Public Health are enrolled onto a funded degree (and effectively paid to study). I completed the Master's of Global Health Science at the University of Oxford (which is broadly equivalent to a Master's in Public Health). With a truly global faculty and inspirational seminars from some of the greats of public health and medicine (Professor Sir Richard Peto and Sir Muir Gray, to name a couple), it really expanded my horizons. It also provided sound training for the gruelling and not to be underestimated Part 1 paper of the Membership of Faculty of Public Health examinations, which I fortunately passed, gaining the Part 2 oral exam and full membership in my second year of training.[vii]

In my third year, I applied for the UK Field Epidemiology Training Programme (FETP), a two-year fellowship addressing competencies in outbreak control, surveillance, applied research and scientific communication, and teaching and training. I was successful and was seconded to Public Health England (PHE) (the health protection remit of which passed to the successor agency, the UKHSA, in 2021), starting training in 2016 with the Centre for Radiation, Chemical and Environmental Hazards (CRCE) Environmental Epidemiology team, and Thames Valley Health Protection Team. I had a key role helping to deliver on national-level projects – for example, the 2018 report on water fluoridation and health, and implementing a new lead-poisoning surveillance system. Locally and regionally, I worked on outbreak investigation and also research on the causes of delays to TB patients gaining a diagnosis and starting treatment.

There were wider opportunities too: FETP training was run alongside its European counterpart programme (European Programme for Intervention Epidemiology Training, EPIET), overseen by the European Centre for Disease Prevention and Control in Stockholm. This meant many of the training modules were conducted across Europe, so I travelled a lot and made many friends from across the continent's public health institutes. I was also fortunate enough to be deployed for a short time to support teaching and training on the Public Health MSc at the University of Sierra Leone, Freetown. The diploma undoubtedly gave me skills and opportunities that would be hard to come by elsewhere.

Posts held and contribution during the pandemic

Towards the end of my training and following the FETP Fellowship, I was able to orient my training placements to my interests (and a later job application) in health protection. This is the field of public health responsible for protecting the public from infectious diseases and non-infectious environmental hazards and threats. Firstly, with our regional CRCE Environmental Hazards and Emergencies team, I learnt a lot with a great team about the first principles of responding to chemical incidents and environmental hazards, including role playing in major incident exercises. With the same team, I led work to review the blood lead concentration in children at which public health teams should take public health action, which led to a lowering of the level.

I then moved to a placement in Colindale, the home of many of the UKHSA's (at that time, Public Health England) specialist infectious disease laboratories and epidemiology teams. It is at the leading edge of communicable disease control in Europe and I was fortunate to be able to work with a number of teams there, particularly the national immunisation team to finalise their health equity audit and related strategy, and the HIV and sexually transmitted infections (STIs) team investigating the risk of a strain of Chlamydia first found elsewhere in Europe that was able to evade detection by the main testing platforms in use in England at the time due to a gene mutation.

I had been back from parental leave for just a few months when the COVID-19 pandemic erupted. I had been doing extra shifts supporting the health protection team to respond to cases and outbreaks, but was not yet otherwise directly involved in the pandemic response. That all changed when my training programme director called to discuss a consultant 'acting up' role to lead on shaping the COVID-19 response in the South East health protection teams. For a year, I worked closely with the health protection teams, local authorities and national specialist technical teams to ensure our COVID-19 response in the South East kept pace with wider developments. This included recruitment to more than double the size of our team, implementing completely new data and surveillance platforms and systems, and sometimes daily changes to guidance and policy. The experience taught me the importance of leadership, management, strategic approach, and how to manage and communicate change well.

I then moved into a more traditional consultant in health protection role to get a better experience of managing incidents and outbreaks (and the non-COVID-19 case load we still had to manage alongside the pandemic) and working with local stakeholders like universities and prisons, and alongside public health colleagues in local government. Subsequently, I successfully applied for a permanent consultant in health protection post with the same team and have been in the role since.

What I enjoy about my current role: the challenges and rewards

I think the best things about my current role are the sheer variety of the challenges faced, the varying pace of work and the great team spirit. There isn't really a typical day in health protection: one day, I can be leading our acute response team managing the public health response to a university student with meningitis, or supporting a care home to safely look after residents during a COVID-19 outbreak. Another day, I might be chairing a case conference risk assessing the potential sources of exposure of a child with lead poisoning, or participating in an exercise testing the public health response to a chemical release (or even responding to the real thing).

New incidents or situations can develop quickly and unpredictably, both locally and of course internationally: infectious diseases such as Zika, COVID-19 and Mpox are either emerging or expanding into new host populations, and older infectious diseases such as measles may re-emerge or cause sporadic outbreaks. You have to be able to cope with change and uncertainty, and a large part of that comes from working within a well-oiled response framework with a supportive team. But there is also more strategic work; for example, I have a particular interest in developing how health protection teams address health equity in their work, and I chair a national network of health protection team health equity leads who recognise we will struggle to realise disease control and elimination goals if we do not address the particular prevention needs of vulnerable people and populations.

How I maintain a work/life balance

During the COVID-19 pandemic, particularly early on, health protection staff worked incredibly hard to help protect our communities. But the long hours and difficult work came at a cost, leading to burnout and emotional fatigue, an outcome from which I wasn't entirely immune. Many individuals and teams in health protection have reflected on the importance of fostering a work/life balance and how that is meaningfully achieved by a team ethos that guards against working overly long hours, senior leaders who respond to the concerns of their staff and flexible working arrangements (I spend one day a week caring for my son).

My ambitions or aspirations for the future

After a year in my first consultant post, I have established myself within the health protection team and wider organisation. You have to get used to the pace of work as a consultant and the time taken to do so shouldn't be underestimated, but I am now starting to think about aspirations for the future. I am fortunate that my job allows me to pursue my professional interests within my core role (for example, applying the health equity agenda within health protection work), but if an opportunity came to do so within 'portfolio' working, so I could work both in health protection and in a separate, perhaps sub-specialist role over different parts of the working week, then I would certainly consider it.

My advice for the next generation

For those pondering whether to work in public health, I would say it is never too late to consider, and prior professional and healthcare experience is often of value. However, if you are a clinician, once you have left patient-facing work, it is not always straightforward to return if you change your mind. If you are unsure at all, spending some time working in a non-patient-facing role may help. Public health is also an unusual medical specialty, in that applicants are welcomed from allied health and non-clinical backgrounds; health protection is no exception and benefits from these diverse skills and experiences, such as environmental health, health policy and analytical skills.

Whatever your background, entrance to public health specialty training is very competitive, so you will need to plan to gain experience and demonstrate commitment to be a successful applicant.[viii] Once you have entered training (or perhaps are pursuing a portfolio route to specialist registration), one of the great things about public health is the flexibility, which means you can really shape your training to your needs and interests (once you have completed membership exams). Even better, you can pursue both a public health career and a rewarding personal and family life, provided you and your employer take active steps to achieve it.

Oluwakemi Olufon, Principal Health Protection Practitioner, UKHSA

What brought me into public health

When describing my journey into public health, I always tell people public health found me. In 2009, I was part of a medical team that travelled to Nairobi offering medical aid to those living in the most impoverished areas of the city. The experience made me value the NHS and our current health systems, but also raised many questions regarding the determinants of health, and the health disparities between low-, middle- and high-income countries. I always knew I wanted to work in the healthcare field and wanted to find the answers to some of my questions, so I completed a BSc in Adult Nursing, and as part of my BSc I had the opportunity to complete an overseas placement. I enrolled in a Public Health Internship in Chicago, where I had my first introduction to the fundamental principles of public health. During the internship, I was able to work with key leaders and political figures and gained a deeper understanding of how public health decisions are made and prioritised for local districts.

I also had the opportunity to work with the Director of Nursing, who supervised my research on childhood obesity in which I received the Investigator Education Certificate. I also assisted the Director of Public Health in updating local policy on how to support mothers from underserved communities with alcohol and substance addiction. The internship was an invaluable experience and enabled me to develop my understanding of the nurse's role within public health. Both international experiences were extremely valuable and shaped my knowledge on public health and community nursing, whether in a slum village in Nairobi or a busy city like Chicago, the principles of public health nursing remained the same:

- to prioritise people;
- to practise effectively;
- to preserve safety; and
- to promote trust.

Training

After completing my BSc, my first nursing role was as a neurosurgery nurse in a busy London hospital, delivering evidence-based, high-quality and individualised patient care. While on one of my first night shifts, I remember discussing my passion for public health and particularly public health nursing with the doctor on call. He would go on to advise me to study for an MSc in Public Health and that the best place to do this was at the London School of Hygiene and Tropical Medicine (LSHTM). At the time, I didn't know how competitive LSHTM was, but was pleasantly surprised when I was offered a place on the MSc Public Health course. The course taught me the fundamental skills and principles needed in public health, such as basic statistics, epidemiology, health promotion and the control of infectious diseases, which to this day I continue to use in my role as a Health Protection Nurse. The content of my MSc course confirmed that health protection and communicable disease control were my key areas of interest within public health, and I continued to develop my knowledge in this area.

Health protection roles

While studying for my MSc, I wanted to accompany my studies with a public health role and became a Community Public Health Nurse in a London borough, specialising in the prevention of childhood illnesses and vaccine-preventable diseases. I provided health advice to parents with children under the age of 5 and led Child Health Clinics across the borough, administering childhood vaccinations, and offering advice to parents on the prevention of childhood illness and injury. My role also included the monitoring and surveillance of children attending local A&E departments and offering additional assistance to families.

Once I completed my MSc and gained experience in Community Public Health Nursing, to further my career I wanted to gain public health experience at local authority level and became an Assistant Public Health Strategist for a London borough. My overall responsibility was to support public health programmes that promote behaviour change, reduce health inequalities and improve the health outcomes of the population. I supported the procurement and contract management of services such as Stop Smoking and assessed the health needs of the local population.

A key achievement while working as a strategist was how I was able to successfully launch the *Active Lives: Active Travel Programme*, which included promoting sustainable travel through implementing the NHS Cycling Strategy and Walking Challenge. Due to the success of the initiative, the borough received Silver Accreditation from NHS London and I gave a lecture about the effectiveness of the initiative to leading public health figures at the Annual NHS Travel Network Conference at City Hall.

What I enjoy about my role

I've always had a passion for health protection and when a role as a Health Protection Nurse became available within the Health Protection Agency (now the UKHSA), I knew it would be my dream job. I have now worked in the health protection field for 12 years and have successfully progressed in my career as a Health Protection Nurse. I enjoyed being the expert lead for gastrointestinal illnesses and have managed several local outbreaks, as well as complex incidents. I also enjoy supporting epidemiological studies and writing formal outbreak reports, and some of my key achievements are publications in both the *British Medical Journal* (BMJ) and *The Lancet*.

My contribution to key public health issues

I have seen the organisation I work in transition from the Health Protection Agency, to Public Health England, to what is now the UKHSA, a new organisation created during the COVID-19 pandemic. There have been many challenges and key achievements during my career, but the current environment of responding to a global pandemic while also having to respond to daily health protection issues and complex incidents has been the most challenging.

In my current role as a Principal Health Protection Practitioner, I lead a large team of Contact Tracers and Health Protection Practitioners managing International Travel Contact Tracing, identifying passengers who have been exposed to COVID-19 on international and domestic flights.

This new role has given me the opportunity to develop my leadership skills on a wider scale and has been a pivotal step in my career in health protection. I have had the opportunity to be involved with the strategic planning of the service, engaging with Cabinet Ministers and the Devolved Administrations, ensuring that our response is aligned across the country. I'm involved in senior policy decisions and a key achievement was having the opportunity to represent the UK at the World Health Organization European Region's consultation on the coordinated decision making on international travel measures.

Although my current role is extremely rewarding, one major challenge is having to navigate political environments. Due to the constant change to policy and changes in the response to the pandemic, decisions are sometimes implemented at such a fast pace. Having to keep up with these changes and lead a team has been challenging, but with the support from colleagues I have continued to keep the public's health at the centre of everything I do.

My ambitions/aspirations for the future

I have a passion for public speaking and have had various opportunities to be a guest lecturer and guest speaker at various events and universities. My next career goal would be to become more involved with teaching and training, as well as being actively involved in public health research, to continue to add to the evidence base and support aspiring public health professionals in their careers.

Maintaining a work/life balance

Working in health protection can be quite demanding and having good prioritisation and time-management skills helps to maintain a healthy work/life balance. I try to ensure I set clear boundaries in the workplace by not taking work home and ensuring I take time out during the day for myself. Remaining consistent with a positive balance helps me to stay motivated and enjoy my work, as it can easily become overwhelming if time is not scheduled for myself. The COVID-19 pandemic brought a new way of working, with an introduction to more hybrid working, which has also enabled me to be more disciplined with maintaining a healthy work/life balance.

Advice for the next generation

My journey into public health was serendipitous at times, but was also conventional by completing a BSc and MSc in Public Health. Your path may not be the same as mine, but you can still take the necessary steps to enter the public health field. My advice would be to choose the path that suits you; it is encouraging to see so many other avenues into public health which were not available when I was entering the field. Public Health Apprenticeships offer public health training and on-the-job experiences via placements in various public health disciplines. Obtaining Practitioner registration with the UK Public Health Register may also give you the accreditation required for public health roles,[ix] so it is important to think outside the box when choosing your career path. Public health jobs are not just within government bodies or local authorities; consider what area of public health you are passionate about and you may find roles in non-governmental organisations, charities, universities and local communities. Public health is such a vast field, so enjoy exploring your interests and having a meaningful career that provides job satisfaction and reward.

Notes

  i See Part 4.
 ii See Part 4.
iii Such as the Communicable Disease Surveillance Centre at Public Health Wales or the European Centre for Disease Prevention and Control.
 iv See Part 4.
  v See Part 4 for routes to registration.
 vi See Part 4.
vii The Faculty of Public Health qualifying examinations are now called Part A and Part B.
viii See Part 4.
 ix See Part 4.

References

1. Faculty of Public Health. *Public Health Practitioners*. Available at: www.fph.org. uk/media/3029/fph_ph_practitioner_09_20-v2.pdf.
2. GOV.UK. *Guidance: Public Health Skills and Knowledge Framework (PHSKF)*. Available at: www.gov.uk/government/publications/public-health-skills-and-knowledge-framework-phskf.
3. GOV.UK. *Policy Paper: Modernising Scientific Careers: The UK Way Forward*. Available at: www.gov.uk/government/publications/modernising-scientific-careers-the-uk-way-forward.
4. World Health Organization. *One Health*. Available at: www.who.int/europe/initiatives/one-health#.

6 Academic public health

*Martin McKee; John Ford; Clare Bambra;
Fiona Sim; Jenny Wright*

Introduction to this function

Academic public health professionals teach public health or carry out research to investigate public health issues. Many are active both in research and in teaching the next generations of public health experts. Academics will set up research projects, usually from their bases in universities, typically applying for funding from grant-awarding bodies for research, which could be on such varied issues as obesity, communicable diseases or climate change, and then they publish their findings, which might influence policy or propose topics for further research. Research in public health tackles some of the most challenging dilemmas facing the health and wellbeing of societies in the UK and internationally. It often contains elements of what are known as both quantitative and qualitative research. In recent decades, research on the impacts of tobacco use, food, air pollution and infectious diseases, for example, has contributed to major changes in health and social policy. Without well-planned research studies and the peer-reviewed published articles that followed, many of the health gains in the population would not have been possible. Academics engaged in modelling and in epidemiological studies on virus transmission, and public health research about behaviour change, as well as those engaged in vaccine development, have been particularly prominent and critically important in establishing the evidence of what works or doesn't work during the COVID-19 pandemic.

Challenges and opportunities – vision for academic public health

*Martin McKee, Professor of European Public Health, London
School of Hygiene and Tropical Medicine*

Public health is different from many academic pursuits. It is done with a purpose: to improve the health of our populations. Generating knowledge is important, but it is secondary to the main goal. It is multidisciplinary. It draws on many disciplinary perspectives, but has no time for those who see

DOI: 10.4324/9781003433699-8

development of their individual discipline as the most important thing. It seeks answers to big questions, using whatever methods are most appropriate rather than rejecting anything that can't be established in a randomised controlled trial. But above all, it is about making a difference. And that means answering the questions that people need to make decisions. The people in question may be the parent deciding whether it is safe to send their child to school in a pandemic, the city mayor deciding whether to build cycle paths, the finance minister deciding whether to increase alcohol taxes or the prime minister deciding how to respond to signs of an emerging health crisis.

I spent late 2020 and early 2021 as a Commissioner, and chair of the Scientific Advisory Board, of the Pan European Commission on Health and Sustainable Development. Chaired by former Italian Prime Minister and European Commissioner Mario Monti, few of my fellow commissioners were from the health field. Instead we had former presidents and prime ministers, bankers and experts from other fields, such as food policy. Our task was to make recommendations about how the world could be better prepared for future threats. I would like to think that we have set an agenda for academic public health in the decades to come.

Our perspective is very broad. We start with 'One Health',[i] the interrelationship between the health of humans, animals and the natural environment, where many of the greatest threats, including COVID-19, arise.

We then move out to consider planetary health, looking at how we prepare for those things we cannot prevent, like the volcanic eruption that recently devastated Tonga, or an asteroid strike, such as that featured in the movie 'Don't Look Up'. But we also look at the threats we can prevent, if the political will exists, such as global heating, deforestation and loss of biodiversity.

We move on to look at the things that either help or harm our pursuit of health. We begin with the usual concerns of public health, like peace, food and shelter. But we update them, including the policies that have left so many people living precarious lives, their struggle to achieve access to justice and, in an increasingly online world, information. We also update the threats, such as organised crime and corruption and those who produce harmful commodities.

Over a century ago, Rudolf Virchow[ii] showed us that public health and politics were inextricably linked. Many of the solutions to the threats to our health can only be tackled through the political process. But this calls upon us in academic public health to speak truth to power. And this is something I've been doing in another role, as a member of Independent SAGE,[iii] listening to the concerns of those affected by COVID-19 and helping their voices be heard. Speaking out may not be easy. Indeed, it is sometimes dangerous. But if we fail to do so, we really should ask whether we would be better doing something else.

Overview of the academic public health function

John Ford, Senior Clinical Lecturer in Health Equity, Wolfson Institute of Population Health, Queen Mary University, London

Description of the function

The two bookends of public health are evidence and communication. Every public health professional works with evidence and data to guide decision-making. Research involves the discovery of new information or evidence, and therefore some of what every public health professional does involves researching their population and ways to improve or protect health. This may involve analysing quantitative data or gathering 'softer' data through discussion groups with different organisations or members of the public. This type of research is one end of the spectrum; at the other end are research studies which are carefully planned using robust methods and are conducted over months and years. Academic public health is, although not exclusively, concerned with this latter type of research.

Some universities have large public health teams which undertake a wide programme of research and teaching, while others have much smaller teams and it is not unusual for there to be only one public health-trained academic in a department. The split between research and teaching varies depending on the individual and university needs. Some public health academics are employed purely to undertake teaching – for example, running a Master's programme. While unusual, some public health academics only undertake research, but most would supervise Master's or PhD students as a minimum.

Contribution to public health issues

Public health research has underpinned the greatest public health achievements in history. The discovery of vaccines and their roll-out through vaccine campaigns has led to dramatic falls in death and disease across the world from many infections, including diphtheria, tetanus, polio, measles, mumps, rubella, meningitis, pertussis and H. influenzae B. The rapid development and delivery of COVID-19 vaccines has prevented millions of deaths worldwide.

Academics have also tracked the continuing rise of deaths and disease from cardiovascular disease (including heart attacks and strokes) in both developed and developing countries. In addition to calling attention to this, academics have researched the causes (for example high blood pressure, obesity) and the so-called 'causes-of-the-causes' (for example, lack of exercise, poor diet and smoking), which are in turn influenced by factors such as marketing by tobacco companies and, conversely, by tobacco control policies. Unpicking the complex web of factors that influence health is one of the challenges and joys of academic life as a public health professional.

The ultimate aim of academic public health is to produce new knowledge that is then implemented and results in changes that improve health.

Sometimes it is possible to demonstrate this success: a team at Bristol University headed by Professor Peter Fleming and Dr Pete Blair were interested in the causes of Sudden Infant Death Syndrome (SIDS), also known as cot death, a devastating tragedy for the infant and family. In the 1980s, they conducted surveys and found that sleeping face down, being covered in too many blankets and passive smoking all increased the chances of a baby's sudden death.[1] These findings were surprising at the time and the researchers needed to conduct more rigorous research to back up their claims. By 1989, their case was strong enough to approach the government's health advisers.[2] After a trial to test the advice in practice, the government launched the 'Back to Sleep' campaign, which advised parents to sleep their babies on their backs. After two years, the number of cot deaths in the UK fell by 70 per cent[3] and, by 2012, the research has been estimated to have prevented 10,000 deaths in the UK and 100,000 worldwide.[4]

While this example shows the power to do good that is inherent to public health research, it also shows that even when the risk factor is something quite simple (whether to place the child on their front or back), it can take many years before research is translated into policy change as we have to be sure that the findings are correct and that the resulting policies themselves are effective.

However, not all risk factors are as simple as the way babies sleep. Alcohol consumption is an increasingly recognised public health challenge and research into its effects and determinants is increasing. While it is clear that alcohol consumption increases the risk of a range of health effects (for example, cardiovascular disease, cancers and liver diseases) and social effects (for example, domestic violence, anti-social behaviour, rape, other crimes and work absenteeism), we have been slow to address these problems through effective public health policies. This is in part because alcohol policies are affected by many more factors than just research findings – for example, alcohol consumption is an accepted part of society and generally enjoys public support. Also, the alcohol industry is a major employer and supports the UK economy, so strategies to reduce harmful alcohol consumption are likely to impact on industry profits and may reduce tax revenue. These are just a few points that policy-makers need to consider when determining an alcohol strategy, and that researchers need to understand when themselves lobbying for their research findings.

So, academia operates in the real world. Its research findings will be challenged, its recommendations will be tested and its voice will have to be heard among other, sometimes competing, interests. Nevertheless, research by public health academics has saved millions of lives and improved the health and wellbeing of many more. And it will continue to do so.

Roles and career opportunities

It is possible to undertake research in most organisations that a public health specialist may find themselves in. However, without dedicated research time and support, it can often be an uphill struggle to get research to a stage of being published in an academic journal. In part, this is because journals are increasing looking for larger multi-centre studies, rather than small local studies.

Therefore, most people who undertake academic public health are employed by a university, or at a minimum have a contractual affiliation to one. The role and responsibilities of an academic public health professional varies from research, teaching, supervising others' research and other academic activities, such as grant reviewing, journal editing and university management. Some academic public health posts are predominantly focused on the design and delivery of teaching, such as within a medical school, whereas others are focused chiefly on research. Public health teaching posts involve more than delivering lectures and seminars. In fact, most time may be spent designing curricula and assessments, coordinating, inviting lecturers and seminar leads, meeting with students who are struggling or building links with the wider university and beyond to potential employers of their graduates.

For those public health academics who spend most of their time doing research, their working lives are generally dominated by applying for grants, managing grants, writing papers and supervision of students. There are several large research grant-giving organisations in the UK, but with success rates usually less than 20% and sometimes as low as 5%, public health academics need a thick skin to deal with rejection. Grant proposals are a significant undertaking: not only do they need a multi-disciplinary team, often across different universities, but they also need engagement with patients and members of the public, a background literature review and detailed costings. Through grant income, the university can cover salary costs, while also developing its reputation for research.

Public health academics are also involved in many other activities which support the wider academic community. These may include reviewing grant applications or sitting on grant-awarding committees, peer-reviewing journal articles or being a journal editor, and supporting the organisation of conferences or networking events and university management, such as managing an academic unit.

Skills and qualifications needed

The key qualification for a permanent academic post is a PhD or Doctor of Medicine (MD).[iv] While this is not always the case, it is much harder to craft an academic career without one. Most people find that a Master's degree is good training and helps them obtain a PhD. However, a PhD, or MD alone, will not guarantee anyone an academic position: universities look for a range of other skills.

Self-motivation and independence are important skills because research requires one or more individuals to drive the research project forward. Many a good research project has been unsuccessful because barriers or challenges have become too difficult. Universities often look at an individual's record of journal article publications or grants to assess whether or not this is the type of person that can push on to complete a research project.

Being able to collaborate and work with a range of different people is another important skill. Research is a team game and needs people with complementary skills. A public health research project may include statisticians, qualitative researchers, health economists, administrators, doctors, members of the public and data managers. Some of these people may be in the same university, while others may be across the country or even the world.

Finally, being able to write concisely and coherently is important, because much of an academic's time is spent writing grant applications, study protocols, papers and editorials. For some people, this comes naturally, but for many others this is a lifelong area of development.

Getting into academic public health

The opportunities for academic training are more formalised for those from a medical background. The General Medical Council stipulates that every medical school programme must include the opportunity for students to spend time exploring an area of their own interest. Many students take this opportunity to undertake a research project with an established academic. After graduation, there is now a formal academic training path. But this was not always the case. Historically, junior doctors who were interested in research had to squeeze research projects into their evenings and weekends. This changed in 2005 with the publication of the Walport Report, which recommended a structured academic training so that junior doctors had dedicated time to develop academic skills.[5]

There is now an Academic Foundation Programme (AFP) for newly qualified doctors to link up with an established academic and have four months of their first two years as doctors dedicated to research. This gives the junior doctor an opportunity to experience the academic world and undertake their own research or contribute to a larger study. The AFP also gives junior doctors opportunities to participate in teaching within a university setting through, for example, leading seminars.

At the point of specialising in public health, junior doctors can apply for an Academic Clinical Fellowship (ACF). These posts are like other public health training posts, but they protect 25% of the junior doctor's time for research in an established university. This may be one or two days a week or a block of three months every year. This Fellowship lasts up to three years and is an opportunity for the individual to undertake research and decide if they would like to undertake a PhD. While in some medical specialities, such as General Practice, ACFs are encouraged to use this time to undertake a Master's degree, most public health training programmes already include a Master's programme at the start.

For those who would like to do a PhD and are successful in obtaining funding or a funded PhD, they can take time out of the training programme to complete their PhD. Following completion of a PhD, many people complete their training through a clinical lecturer position which allows 50% of their time to be protected for research. Finally, after all this training, an individual may be appointed to a permanent academic position.

While this is the formal training pathway, in truth few public health academics follow this route. Some will not have undertaken the AFP, ACF or clinical lectureship, but most will have undertaken a PhD or MD at some stage. For example, some people enter medicine after having completed a PhD.

The pathway to academic public health for people coming from backgrounds other than medicine is less structured and, arguably, more difficult. Some people may already have a PhD before entering public health training or may have already been employed as a researcher within a university. While some of the opportunities mentioned above are restricted to those with a medical background (such as AFP and ACF), it is not to say that there are not opportunities. Most public health programmes will facilitate an academic placement at a university and there are similar PhD opportunities. Increasingly, training programmes are trying to address the disparities in academic training opportunities between those from a medical background and those not.

Why this has been a rewarding career

Having been involved in research for the past 15 years and worked across three different universities, academic public health is a great job. First and foremost, I have a deep personal connection to my area of academic interest, health inequalities, and I am grateful to have a job which so closely aligns with my personal values and beliefs. There is also a large amount of freedom in academic public health – we get to choose what areas to research and who to collaborate with. However, the greatest possible reward is the knowledge that through research we have the potential to make huge improvements to health, wellbeing and society at large.

It is not uncommon for academics to continue to work after retirement, even though they do not get paid for it. Few other organisations have employees who continue to work free of charge after retirement simply because they love what they do.

Career story

Clare Bambra, Professor of Public Health, Newcastle University

How I got started in public health

Academic public health is an exciting and varied discipline, with colleagues working together from across a variety of disciplines using a diversity of research methods. On a daily basis, I get the chance to work with sociologists, nutritionists, epidemiologists, health economists, historians, biologists, economists, geographers and health policy experts. This diversity is reflected in my own career path.

I studied political science as an undergraduate at the University of Birmingham, graduating BSocSc in 1998. I then went on to do a Master's and a PhD in public policy at the University of Manchester, finishing my PhD in 2002. My PhD examined social policy and health care systems across Europe.

I started looking for a job towards the end of my PhD and I was attracted to an opportunity in the Department of Public Health at the University of Liverpool. This was a two-year post as a post-doctoral researcher. I was fortunate enough to get the job – working on a systematic review of the impacts of 'welfare to work' policies on the health and employment in Europe of people with a long-term health condition or disability. My line manager at Liverpool was Dame Professor Margaret Whitehead, the W.H. Duncan Professor of Public Health and a world-leading expert in health inequalities.

When I first joined the Department of Public Health at Liverpool, I had no idea what public health was! Like many researchers trained in political science and health policy, I only understood health as health services and the NHS. So my time in Liverpool taught me about public health as a wider subject and notably the role of social, economic and political factors in shaping the health of the public. I benefited from the expertise at Liverpool and also from various training courses in public health research methods, such as epidemiology. Working alongside Dame Professor Margaret Whitehead and other seminal colleagues who were working at Liverpool at the time – such as Dr Alex Scott Samuel and Professor Simon Capewell – I learned about health inequalities, and how health differs by gender, ethnicity, socio-economic status (deprivation, education, employment, income, class) and other aspects of social identity.

What brought me to public health

So, this early period at Liverpool launched my career in public health and gave me a passion for understanding and reducing health inequalities in the UK and beyond.

Socio-economic inequalities in health mean that people with higher incomes and occupational status (for example, professionals such as doctors, teachers or lawyers) generally have better health outcomes and higher life expectancies than those with lower incomes or occupational status (for example, shop workers, cleaners or call centre workers).[6] There are also geographical inequalities in health. For example, Americans live three years less than their counterparts in France or Sweden. People in the north of England live more than two years less than those in the south and there is a nine-year gap in life expectancy between the most and least deprived neighbourhoods in the UK.[7] Gender also matters for health – in the UK, men have lower life expectancies than women, but women spend their extra years with higher levels of ill health.[8] There are also considerable inequalities in health by ethnicity, with British Asian and British Black citizens having lower life expectancies than White British citizens.[9] These different social categories (for example, socio-economic status, gender, ethnicity – as well as other aspects of social identity, such as sexuality) are experienced collectively, leading to complex intersectional experiences of social inequalities in health.[10]

Health inequalities are systematic and unfair and so finding out how we can reduce them has been the focus of my public health research career. Given my original training in political science and public policy, my work has had a particular focus on the role of social and economic policies in shaping health inequalities.

In 2004, after my two-year post-doctoral post at the University of Liverpool ended, I moved to Sheffield to take up a Lectureship in Social Policy at Sheffield Hallam University. Here, I was able to continue my research into health inequalities in Europe and I also benefited from undertaking teaching at both undergraduate and postgraduate levels. I also obtained a Postgraduate Certificate in Higher Education during my time at Sheffield Hallam. In 2005, I was lucky enough to move to the North East, which had been a long-term personal goal. I was appointed as Lecturer in Public Health Policy at Durham University, working alongside eminent colleagues such as Professor David Hunter (a prominent scholar of health policy) and Professor Sarah Curtis (a leading health geographer). I then spent the next 12 years at Durham University and was promoted to Professor there, in the Geography Department, in 2010. During my time at Durham University, I also spent three years as the Executive Director of the Wolfson Research Institute for Health and Wellbeing, which was an exciting interdisciplinary organisation. At Durham University, I was able to expand the intellectual basis of my research – learning from colleagues about geographical and public health policy approaches to health inequalities. This significantly shaped my thinking and research focus. In 2017, I was appointed as Professor of Public Health in Newcastle University's Population Health Sciences Institute in the Faculty of Medical Sciences.

What I enjoy about my current role: the challenges and rewards

I am currently Professor of Public Health, Population Health Sciences Institute, Faculty of Medical Sciences, Newcastle University, UK. This is an extremely challenging but also really rewarding role. I lead a large multidisciplinary research group, with colleagues from a diversity of backgrounds, experiences and disciplines, including sociology, criminology, economics, anthropology, geography, pharmacy, public health and epidemiology. Together, we work on a variety of different research projects examining health inequalities in the North East, the UK, Europe and globally.

The challenges for me come from managing my research projects, staff and students and ensuring that all our work is delivered on time and to a high standard. However, the rewards of public health research are much higher. By working with a diversity of colleagues, there is a stimulating exchange of ideas and perspectives. In my work, every day is different as I work across a variety of research projects, in multiple project teams consisting of different people from Newcastle University and other UK universities, as well as global collaborations with international scholars.

At Newcastle University, I am able to teach a variety of different students, both clinical and non-clinical, at undergraduate and postgraduate levels. This includes teaching health inequalities and public health to our undergraduate medicine, pharmacy and biomedical sciences students. At the postgraduate level, I contribute to our Master's in Public Health programme, which attracts students from across the world. I also supervise several PhD students whose projects focus on health inequalities.

Another important and valued part of my current post is the close connection I have with public health policy-makers and practitioners in local and national government, international agencies such as the European Commission and the World Health Organization, and charitable organisations and policy think-tanks. This partnership working with colleagues outside academia has always been an exciting part of public health research, and it also means that my work remains relevant to current priorities – most notably COVID-19.

My contribution to key public health issues and COVID-19

At the time of writing, the omicron strain of COVID-19 has reignited the global pandemic. Over the last three years, I have been focusing my work on the impact of the COVID-19 pandemic on health inequalities – arguing that it is a 'syndemic pandemic' (see below).[11]

COVID-19 deaths are twice as high in the most deprived neighbourhoods of England than in the most affluent, they are higher in the more deprived regions (Figure 6.1) and also in urban compared to rural areas.[12] There are also significant inequalities by ethnicity and race, with the mortality among people from ethnic minorities in the UK considerably higher than expected.

In our report, *A Year of COVID-19 in the North*,[13] we found that during the first year of the pandemic (March 2002 to February 2021), London (264.8 per 100,000), the North West (233.7 per 100,000), West Midlands (214 per 100,000) and the North East (212.8 per 100,000) had the highest COVID-19 mortality rates (Figure 6.1). In contrast, the South West

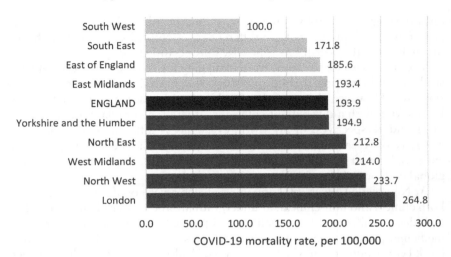

Figure 6.1 Regional COVID-19 mortality rates per 100,000 (March 2020 to March 2021) (reproduced with permission from Munford *et al.*, 2021)

(100.0 per 100,000) and the South East (171.8 per 100,000) had the lowest COVID-19 mortality rates.

In our research, we found that this is because of the interaction of the pandemic with existing social, economic and health inequalities: COVID-19 is a 'syndemic pandemic'.[14] The concept of a *syndemic* was originally derived from understanding the relationships between HIV/AIDS, substance use and violence in the USA in the 1990s.[15] A syndemic exists when risk factors or co-morbidities are intertwined, interactive and cumulative – that is, when multiple causes of ill health pile upon and reinforce one another in ways that make illness from COVID-19 more common and more damaging.[16] In our research, we have argued that for the most disadvantaged communities, COVID-19 is experienced as a syndemic – a co-occurring, synergistic pandemic which interacts with and exacerbates existing chronic health and social conditions (Figure 6.2).

Beyond the pandemic, my main contribution to public health research has been using my diverse disciplinary background to highlight the importance of political and economic policies for health inequalities. For example, I led a large Leverhulme Trust grant that explored the impacts of austerity on health inequalities in England.[17] I have also evaluated how the 2000–2010 National Health Inequalities Strategy in England reduced geographical inequalities in health.[18] Currently, I am co-leading a large National Institute for Health Research (NIHR) grant examining the impacts of the Universal Credit welfare policy on inequalities in mental health,[19] and I also lead a large Wellcome Trust grant that explores the 'north–south' health divide in this country.[20]

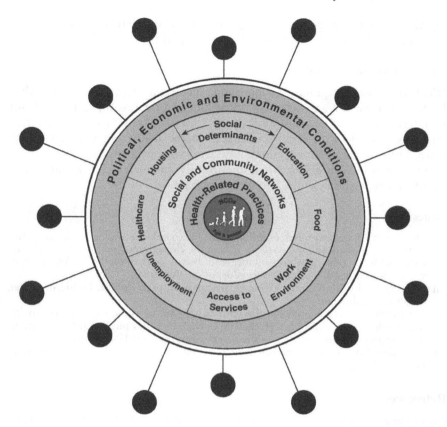

Figure 6.2 The syndemic of COVID-19, non-communicable diseases (NCDs) and the social determinants of health (reproduced with permission from Bambra *et al.*, 2020)

Maintaining a work/life balance

I use various techniques to enable me to have a work/life balance. These include being very strict about my working hours, ensuring that I take regular breaks – including a lunch break (which unfortunately is a declining trend in UK universities!), seldom working on weekends, and I also don't have a smart phone, so that I can prevent myself from accessing emails outside of office hours! My productivity has remained just as high as when I did longer hours – in fact, research shows that working long hours does not improve quality or quantity, particularly for creative intellectual work such as research.

My aspirations for the future

My aspirations for the future remain the same as they always have been – to use research evidence to help reduce health inequalities. I want to ensure that my work remains relevant to current policies and debates in public health and to train the next generation of health inequalities researchers.

Advice for the next generation

Whatever your disciplinary background, there is a place for you in public health research! It's an extremely rewarding and interesting career and one that has never been more important or topical. My advice is to work as much as possible with senior colleagues in the field from whom you can learn, but also network and collaborate with your peers as they will be with you throughout your career. Most importantly, pursue an area within public health research about which you are passionate.

Notes

  i One Health is an integrated, unifying approach to balance and optimise the health of people, animals and ecosystems. It uses the close, interdependent links among these fields to create new surveillance and disease control methods. Available at: www.who.int/news-room/fact-sheets/detail/one-health#.
 ii A German physician, anthropologist, pathologist, prehistorian, biologist, writer, editor and politician.
iii Independent SAGE is a group of scientists who are working together to provide independent scientific advice to the UK government and public on how to minimise deaths and support Britain's recovery from the COVID-19 crisis.
 iv Note that MD denotes a higher degree in medicine in the UK; it does not imply first qualification as in some countries.

References

1. Fleming, P.J., Gilbert, R., Azaz, Y., Berry, P.J., Rudd, P.R., Stewart, A. and Hall, E. Interaction between bedding and sleeping position in the sudden infant death syndrome: A population based case-control study. *British Medical Journal*, 301(6743): 85–9, 1990.
2. Bristol Health Partners. *Cot Deaths: Saving More than 100,000 Young Lives Worldwide*. Available at: www.bristolhealthpartners.org.uk/news/cot-deaths-saving-more-than-100000-young-lives-worldwide/.
3. Office for National Statistics. *Health Statistics Quarterly* (Winter). The Stationery Office, 70, 2004.
4. Blair, P.S., Sidebotham, P., Berry, P.J., Evans, M. and Fleming, P.J. Major epidemiological changes in sudden infant death syndrome: A 20-year population-based study in the UK. *The Lancet*, 367:314–19, 2006; Mitchell, E.A. and Blair, P.S. SIDS prevention: 3000 lives saved but we can do better. *New Zealand Medical Journal*, 2012; Dattani, N. and Cooper, N. Trends in cot death. *Health Statistical Quarterly* (Spring). Office of National Statistics, The Stationery Office, 10–16, 2000.
5. *Report of the Academic Sub-Committee of the Modernising Medical Careers and the UK Cancer Research Collaboration March 2005*. Available at: www.ukcrc.org/wp-content/uploads/2014/03/Medically_and_Dentally-qualified_Academic_Staff_Report.pdf.
6. Eikemo, T.A., Bambra, C., Huijts, T., and Fitzgerald, R. The European Social Survey (ESS) rotating module on the social determinants of health: The first

pan-European sociological health inequalities survey, *European Sociological Review*, 3: 137–153, 2017.

7. Bambra, C. *Health Divides: Where You Live Can Kill You*, Bristol, Policy Press, 2016.
8. Bambra, C., Albani, V. and Franklin, P. Covid-19 and the gender health paradox. *Scandinavian Journal of Public Health*, 49: 17–26, 2021.
9. Nazroo, J. and Williams, D. The social determination of ethnic/racial inequalities in health. In *The Social Determinants of Health*, Marmot, M. and R. Wilkinson, R. (eds), Oxford, Oxford University Press, 238–66, 2006.
10. Kapilashrami, A., Hill, S. and Meer, N. What can health inequalities researcher learn from an intersectionality perspective? Understanding social dynamics with an inter categorical approach. *Social Theory & Health*, 13, 288–307, 2015.
11. Bambra, C., Riordan, R., Ford, J. and Matthews, F. The COVID-19 pandemic and health Inequalities. *Journal of Epidemiology and Community Health*, 174: 964–8, 2020.
12. Bambra, C., Lynch, J. and Smith, K.E. *Unequal Pandemic: COVID-19 and Health Inequalities*, Bristol, Policy Press, 2021.
13. Munford, L., Khavandi, S., Bambra, C. *et al. A Year of COVID-19 in the North: Regional Inequalities in Health and Economic Outcomes*, Northern Health Science Alliance, Newcastle, 2021. Available at: www.thenhsa.co.uk/app/uploads/2021/09/A-Year-of-COVID-in-the-North-report-2021.pdf.
14. Bambra *et al.*, 2020, op. cit.
15. Singer, M. *Introduction to Syndemics: A Systems Approach to Public and Community Health*. San Francisco, CA, Jossey-Bass, 2009.
16. Singer M. A dose of drugs, a touch of violence, a case of AIDS: Conceptualizing the SAVA syndemic. *Free Inquiry in Creative Sociology*, 28: 13–24, 2000.
17. Bambra, C. (ed). *Health in Hard Times: Austerity and Health Inequalities*, Bristol, Policy Press, 2019.
18. Robinson, T., Brown, H., Norman, P., Barr, B., Fraser, L. and Bambra, C. Investigating the impact of New Labour's English health inequalities strategy on geographical inequalities in infant mortality: A time trend analysis. *Journal of Epidemiology & Community Health*, 73: 564–8, 2019.
19. Craig, P. and Bambra, C. *Evaluation of the Health Impacts of Universal Credit: A Mixed Methods Study*, NIHR, 2021. Available at: https://fundingawards.nihr.ac.uk/award/NIHR131709.
20. NIHR School for Public Health Research. *Funding Boost to Tackle England's North–South Health Divide*. Available at: www.sphr.nihr.ac.uk/news-and-events/funding-boost-to-tackle-englands-north-south-health-divide/.

7 International and global health

David Heymann; Mala Rao; Leena Inamdar;
Manuelle Hurwitz; Fiona Sim; Jenny Wright

Introduction to this function

This chapter focuses on the well-established contribution made by public health professionals to improving health across national borders, particularly for those in developing or low-income countries. There has been debate in recent years over the distinction between international and global health. 'Global health' is *usually* taken to refer to issues that affect the health of the whole world's population and which require global input and global solutions. 'International health' *usually* refers to health issues identified within, typically, developing countries, as well as issues which require a cooperative approach across national borders.

Public health professionals working in international or global health tend to focus on health programme design and management. This is a particularly challenging but rewarding area of work, where public health skills and experience are used to the full. Activities can include needs assessments, community engagement, planning programmes, fund-raising and managing the delivery of these programmes. Targeted public health projects are effective ways of improving and protecting the health of the population, particularly in low-income countries, where they supplement and enhance services provided by their own governments. The public health workforce must work with great sensitivity to appreciate the cultures, wishes and priorities of communities or governments on both long-term programmes such as setting up and implementing national or local immunisation services or introducing hygienic toilet facilities to a village, to responding to emergency threats to public health, such as an earthquake or an outbreak of a serious communicable disease.

Challenges and opportunities – vision for international and global public health

David Heymann, Professor of Infectious Diseases, London School of Hygiene and Tropical Medicine and Head of the Centre on Global Health Security at Chatham House

We would do well to better listen to what lower- and middle-income countries (LMICs) actually view as priorities before we act in their support.

DOI: 10.4324/9781003433699-9

Industrialised countries in fact risk being too directive in their assistance without truly understanding the priorities of the countries they support. Some African countries during the COVID-19 pandemic have been criticised, for example, for not prioritising vaccination of their populations against COVID-19, because they had other disease priorities that cause more reported deaths, such as malaria. Dialogue with these countries by those that support them, and the international organisations, could in fact result in better outcomes for all.

All countries must develop core public health capacity to detect and respond effectively to infections as and when they occur; this is a requirement of the International Health Regulations, to which all Member States of the World Health Organization (WHO) adhere. The Global Health Security Agenda is a voluntary partnership between industrialised countries and LMICs that provides, along with WHO, an external peer assessment of core public health capacities and supports countries in their development. But, often, when LMICs develop plans based on this evaluation, the plan is not funded as a whole, and donor countries choose to fund only those components of the plan of interest to their own national priorities.

Some LMICs accept support from donor countries without generating their own supplemental resources, especially if the support is not offered for their priorities. The challenge for young public health leaders worldwide is to help shift this paradigm from top-down donor support to support based on LMIC requests and their generation of matched funding for national priorities upwards. More shared responsibility from this paradigm shift will facilitate not only action, but also innovation within their own systems and context. Matched funding requirements of the Global Fund for AIDS, TB and Malaria, and of GAVI, the Global Vaccine Alliance, are a step in this direction.

We have learned from the COVID-19 pandemic that in order to be better prepared for infectious disease outbreaks we need to ensure that three interlocking functions are in place:

- a strong public health workforce to prevent and/or rapidly detect and respond to epidemics, pandemics and endemic disease (prevention measures at the animal/human interface, strong surveillance and detection systems and the capacity to respond rapidly);
- resilient, accessible and sustainable healthcare that can accommodate a surge of patients and continue routine services at the same time; and
- a means of enabling more healthy populations with minimal co-morbidities that can resist infection.

One way forward would be to have an international framework convention as being discussed by WHO, which would encompass these three interlocking functions with requirements at both the national and the international levels, similar to the framework convention on tobacco control.

Another challenge for the future is to promote innovation within the public and private sectors of LMICs. This will involve better collective understanding of how innovation can be promoted and how regulatory systems can be strengthened to evaluate and license rapidly those innovations that are safe and effective.

The public health workforce of the future will need practical experience in working internationally in LMICs, cultural sensitivity, patience and language skills, so field experience should be part of any training programme.

If countries do work together in a way that is collaborative among LMICs and donor countries, there can be major achievements; for example, global solidarity achieved smallpox eradication during the Cold War when technicians from the former USSR and the USA worked closely together despite the political differences of their governments. More recently, neighbouring countries working together enabled permission for polio vaccinators to enter Taliban-controlled areas of Afghanistan, and likewise, fostered days of tranquillity in other countries with disputes, so that polio eradication activities could continue.

When I began my public health career almost 50 years ago, the world population was approximately 3.2 billion. It is now over seven billion. This expansion in population has occurred with increased demand for animal-based foods, causing increases in animal husbandry often near population agglomerations, facilitating the spill-over of animal infections to humans, and is being influenced by such phenomena as climate change and environmental degradation. We must find ways to work differently in such a complicated world. Young public health workers should grasp opportunities to have an impact when they arise. My own first assignments from the US Centers for Disease Control and Prevention (CDC) back in 1976 were to the first known Legionnaires disease outbreak in the USA, followed by the first known outbreak of Ebola haemorrhagic fever in the Democratic Republic of Congo. I was able to participate in the investigation and control of these outbreaks, because I had placed myself in the right place at the right time and was willing to make myself available to participate.

So my message is to get out there where the action is, make yourself available when opportunities arise and make a difference in this world in need of strong public health!

Overview of international and global public health

Mala Rao, Director, Ethnicity and Health Unit, Department of Primary Care and Public Health, Imperial College, London and
Leena Inamdar, Global Health Lead, Head of Programme, New Variant Assessment Platform, Science Group, UK Health Security Agency

Introduction to global public health

There has never been a more fulfilling time to work in global public health than now. COVID-19 has highlighted the importance of the role of public health globally, as well as across the three domains of health protection, health improvement and healthcare public health. Post pandemic, it is evident that public health specialists will be needed not only to ensure better pandemic preparedness and strategies for tackling public health crises such as antimicrobial resistance (AMR), but also to address the health impacts of the rapidly escalating socio-economic inequalities and the climate crisis, for which the pandemic is sometimes described as a dress rehearsal.[1]

What is global public health?

Global health is 'public health somewhere else'.[2] Consequently, global public health practitioners often work in parts of the world with the greatest health needs. The most satisfying aspect of this work is in contributing to positive change. Global public health practitioners are typically involved in health system strengthening[3] and capacity building in low- and middle-income countries. They undertake activities such as health needs assessment, monitoring and evaluation, technical assistance to programmes and supporting policy-making. Global health work is often project-funded either by governments or overseas donors.

Contribution to public health

Global public health encompasses the ideology of societal health equity and aims to reduce unacceptable and avoidable health inequities. Global public health aims to achieve 'Health for All'.[4] The UK was the first country to publish a strategy entitled 'Health is Global – a UK Government Strategy 2008–2013'.[5] It called for five areas of action: health security; strong and fairer systems for health; more effective international health organisations; freer and fairer trade; and strengthening the way we develop and use evidence to improve policy and practice. The UK Aid Strategy 2015[6] committed science and technology funding to tackling global risks such as AMR and climate change. There are reciprocal benefits to the UK by engaging globally, through applying overseas experience to tackle UK health problems. The NHS can learn from resource-poor nations about efficient use of scarce resources. Besides, challenges such as AMR and global warming are not confined to national boundaries and can only be resolved if developed countries support their LMIC partners to take appropriate action.

Public health roles and career opportunities

Global health professionals work across multi-disciplinary fields:

1 *Providing technical assistance and expertise* in non-communicable (NCDs) and communicable diseases – for example, laboratory and surveillance strengthening, data analytics, maternal and child health, mental health and climate-sensitive health risks.

2 *Policy analysis and strategy development* by translation of scientific evidence to influence health policy and national strategies – for example, vaccine policy and national action plans for disaster management.
3 *Programme management and implementation* – for example, Malaria, TB, reproductive health and tobacco control programmes.
4 *Research, teaching and workforce development* for capability building to strengthen health systems.

In future, we will need traditional fields of public health practice and skills in innovative applications of technology driving public health interventions.[7] Future career opportunities are likely to be in:

- *Communicable diseases control, infectious diseases, One Health, AMR, Zoonotic Diseases, pandemic preparedness, health security.* There will be a need for health protection practitioners from disciplines like epidemiology, virology, microbiology, genomics, veterinary science and emergency preparedness.
- *Digital health, modelling outbreak forecasting.* With growing emphasis on pandemic preparedness, public health specialists skilled in data analytics, bioinformatics, geographic information systems, modelling and forecasting, artificial intelligence, robotics and digital health for preventive healthcare will be needed.
- *Allied disciplines* such as behavioural sciences and health economics will be needed to improve acceptability and cost-effectiveness of public health interventions.
- *Non-communicable diseases, mental health, reproductive, maternal, newborn and child health (RMNCH).* With continuing increase in the burden of NCDs, there will be an ongoing need for specialists in lifestyle diseases, mental health and maternal and child health and in health systems strengthening, to enhance the frontline management of these conditions.
- *Planetary Health, Climate and Health, Chemicals, Radiation and Environmental health.* In line with the World Health Day 2022 theme, 'Our Planet, Our Health',[8] there is a growing need for specialists in health, climate change and the environment.

Settings for global public health in the UK and internationally

Global public health practitioners may be based in the UK or overseas.

UK-based

CIVIL SERVICE

In the UK Department of Health and Social Care (DHSC), there are opportunities to work as project officers, policy advisors and heads of teams, leading global health security programmes and bilateral or multilateral engagements such as the G7 and G20. The Office for Health Improvement and Disparities (OHID) has NCD specialists working in global health. The Foreign, Commonwealth and Development Office (FCDO) employs health advisors based in the UK or overseas. Government departments such as the Ministry of Defence or Department for Business, Energy and Industrial Strategy also have opportunities for public health specialists. Government agencies such as the UK Health Security Agency (UKHSA) may offer opportunities through its global health projects.

ACADEMIC PUBLIC HEALTH DEPARTMENTS

Academic public health departments throughout the UK have partnerships with developing countries and can offer opportunities for global public health practitioners in research, teaching, health systems strengthening and capacity building.

NHS AND HEALTH EDUCATION ENGLAND

These have partnerships with international partners for teaching, research and twinning, where public health practitioners may find opportunities to get involved.

NON-GOVERNMENTAL ORGANISATIONS (NGOS) AND CHARITABLE ORGANISATIONS

NGOs such as Médecins Sans Frontières (MSF), Oxfam, Save the Children and Doctors of the World offer exciting career opportunities for public health professionals to work in the UK or overseas in a wide range of roles.

PRIVATE SECTOR

Public health consultancies working on large international projects in collaboration with governments or international NGOs often have opportunities to work in an advisory capacity or in programme implementation.

Overseas

There are opportunities to work in community-based organisations, with national public health institutes, NGOs or in the private sector. Global organisations such as the United Nations Children's Fund (UNICEF), World Health Organization (WHO), Food and Agricultural Organization (FAO) and World Bank also offer attractive careers in policy and strategy development for public health specialists. Global health professionals work nationally, regionally, such as in Africa or Asia, or at the global headquarters of these organisations.

Skills and qualifications required

Working in global health can be hugely satisfying. This experience broadens one's mindset by offering exposure to and learning from different systems and cultures. It can also be challenging to work in unfamiliar and resource-constrained settings.

The key qualifications, skills and attitudes to become successful in a global health career are as follows:

Qualifications

There are no specific qualifications that are recognised as essential to work in global health. However, some qualifications can help launch your career in global health. A Master's in Public Health, Global Health, Health Policy, Global Studies or International Development will give you a good understanding of the global health landscape. Training in bioinformatics, modelling, geographic information systems, health economics, biomedical sciences, genomics, emergency preparedness and field epidemiology are valuable. Qualifications in health promotion, mental health, behavioural sciences and health economics may also be beneficial.

Skills

Global health needs these skills, in line with the UK Public Health Skills and Knowledge Framework:[9]

LEADERSHIP SKILLS

Leadership, influencing and negotiation skills are required when working in policy and strategy, and in senior technical roles which require working with governmental agencies and multilateral organisations.

TECHNICAL SKILLS

These encompass skills in health protection, health improvement, biomedical sciences, surveillance and data analytics, behavioural science and health economics.

PROGRAMME AND PROJECT MANAGEMENT SKILLS

Programme and project management skills and experience are essential for programme implementation. Knowledge of project management tools, monitoring and evaluation and business management are critically important for success in these areas of work.

BUSINESS MANAGEMENT AND ADMINISTRATIVE SKILLS

Skills in business administration, finance, logistics and supply chain management are needed for business support in global health programmes.

Important qualities and attitudes for working in global health

Global public health practitioners need appropriate attitudes and personal qualities such as:

1 resilience and adaptability to work in new, demanding environments and extreme climatic conditions;
2 a willingness to live in locations with poor access to basic amenities such as safe water, hygienic food, good sanitation, electricity, internet or roads;
3 cultural sensitivity to understand the context in which communities live and the ability to build trust when working with diverse populations;
4 a positive mindset and curiosity to find context-specific locally appropriate solutions; and
5 the ability to recognise that there is much that wealthy economies can learn from their LMIC counterparts.

How to enter

Practical experience

There is no substitute for field experience to build your global health career. Look for volunteering and work placements to understand global health. The WHO, United Nations (UN) or charities offer short-term internships and fellowships that will help build your CV and experience. Research online, talk to global health practitioners, read about vacancies at the WHO, the UN and NGOs to understand the skills-set required and identify your specific interest. Find a mentor to support you who can signpost you to relevant opportunities to get you started. If you are successful in being appointed to the national public health specialty training programme,[i] you may be able to undertake a global health placement in one of these organisations, although they are highly sought after and therefore competitive to obtain.

Where public health specialists and practitioners have made a tangible difference

Britain has a proud history of involvement in global public health. It includes leaders from past centuries, such as Sir Ronald Ross. He was a British doctor who won the Nobel Prize for medicine for his discovery of the malarial parasite and how malaria was transmitted, through extensive public health research carried out in India and globally. While the era of striking global life-changing discoveries by individuals may be over, there are many

UK public health specialists whose work, ranging from vaccine discovery and distribution to infectious disease modelling and advocacy against smoking or on the wider determinants of health, is recognised to have helped shift the health improvement and protection dial globally.

Why this function has provided a rewarding career

Leena Inamdar

My post-graduate journey after my medical graduation in India started as a primary care clinician and later continued within public health specialist training in the UK. I specialised in communicable disease control and led front-line outbreak response. After 17 years in the UK, I moved back to India, working with the Ministry of Health and Family Welfare for the introduction of the pneumococcal vaccine nationally. I later joined the US Centers for Disease Control (CDC) India team and led a project to strengthen surveillance of acute encephalitis syndrome in high-risk states, leading to a change in the national guidelines. I have undertaken consultancies as an expert for WHO projects, such as delivering public health leadership training in Kazakhstan. I am currently leading a global programme at the UK Health Security Agency to strengthen genomic surveillance in our partner countries to detect new variants of SARS-CoV-2 and other new and emerging pathogens. From implementing vaccination clinics in local communities to developing national vaccine policy impacting about 27 million infants born in India annually, to strengthening surveillance and diagnostic capacity for infectious diseases, I have worked across all three domains of public health at local, national and global levels. The chance to bring public health interventions to the doorstep of disadvantaged populations drives my passion to work in global health.

Mala Rao

Following nearly three decades in public health in England, initially as a specialist trainee, then in public health practice and policy development in NHS Health Authorities and later at the Department of Health, I had the opportunity under the aegis of the UK 'Health Is Global' strategy to establish the Public Health Foundation of India's first Institute of Public Health as its founding Director from 2008 to 2011. During this period, not only was I able to put my public health specialist skills and training to good use in launching training programmes for research, but I was also able to design development programmes to strengthen the public health skills of district medical officers and other grades of public health specialists and practitioners. Most importantly, I was also able to demonstrate to the state and national governments the value of the Institute in supporting public health policy development by leading research and reviews on topics ranging from improving healthcare quality to the health impacts of climate change. Spurred by the success of this involvement in global health, and the mutual benefits of the shared learning to both India and the UK, I extended my stay in India, at the invitation of the Indian state and national governments, to lead the impact evaluation of health financing innovations and the piloting of new models of primary care. The outcomes of these studies, in terms of policy reforms to improve access to better healthcare, have benefited millions of people in India and encouraged me to accept invitations from other parts of the developing world to help strengthen health systems in their countries. More recently, I have begun to channel my knowledge and experience to support charitable organisations such as WaterAid to achieve their public health goals.

Career story

Manuelle Hurwitz, Director of Global Programmes, International Planned Parenthood Federation

IPPF – background and organisational setup

The International Planned Parenthood Federation (IPPF) is a global provider and a leading advocate of sexual and reproductive health and rights (SRHR) for all. IPPF was born in the early 1950s through the action of a group of activists committed to recognising 'women's right to control their fertility and increase access to family planning services'. Today, IPPF is a federation of 143 autonomous members and collaborative partners, working in over 146 countries and running about 40,000 service points worldwide.[10] Over the years, in line with the International Conference on Population and Development (ICPD) in 1994, IPPF has broadened its mandate beyond contraception to include the full range of sexual and reproductive health and rights, reflecting the definition from the Guttmacher-Lancet Commission (2018).[11] This definition takes a positive approach to sexuality and reproduction by 'recognising the role played by pleasurable sexual relationships, trust and communication in the promotion of self-esteem and overall wellbeing'.

As a global federation, IPPF's action is through local partners working through advocacy, community empowerment and service delivery to address gender inequality and reach marginalised and excluded people, who because of their age, race, socio-economic status, gender identity, sexual orientation, disability, HIV status and other factors see their human and sexual and reproductive rights violated and face barriers in accessing essential care. IPPF engages young people in its governance and programming, seeking to increase their leadership and control over solutions to sexual and reproductive health needs they identified. Programmes delivered by local actors across the world have also allowed IPPF to work across the development and humanitarian nexus, ensuring sustained presence before, during and post crises. IPPF in-country partners in fragile settings have worked in preparedness and strengthened their ability to provide and enable the provision of life-saving sexual and reproductive health services[12] guided by the Minimum Initial Service Package (MISP) for Reproductive Health in Crises.[13]

IPPF works through six regional offices located in Brussels, Nairobi, Tunis, New York, Kuala Lumpur and New Delhi. Together with the London office, these constitute the IPPF Secretariat, with the primary role of serving Member Associations, so that in turn they are able to effectively respond to the sexual and reproductive health and rights needs of local communities. Volunteerism is central to IPPF's ethos and millions of volunteers work with the federation around the world, in governance, in programme implementation and service delivery, and as SRHR advocates.

Sexual and reproductive health and rights – a global perspective

According to the report of the Guttmacher-Lancet Commission (2018),[14] 4.3 billion people of reproductive age worldwide will have inadequate sexual and reproductive health over their lifetime. Many of them – youth, marginalised and crisis-affected populations – fall outside public sector reach or do not use their services.

Each year, 25 million unsafe abortions take place globally. The definition of what constitutes an 'unsafe' abortion was recently revisited by WHO due to the increase in women safely self-managing their abortion through medical abortion drugs.

214 million women and girls in developing regions have an unmet need for modern contraception.[15] A recent review by the Reproductive Health Supplies Coalition shows that more than 80% of contraceptives in LMICs are financed by out-of-pocket expenditures rather than through public sector or donor funding – highlighting a key concern in equity of access to poor and vulnerable groups,[16] but also the role played by service delivery models beyond health facilities to bring services closer to the people. IPPF's current service delivery profile reflects this trend, with 85% of its service delivery points being community-based distributors and through specific partnerships established with associated clinics such as social franchising.

In 2021, an estimated 1.5 million people became newly infected with HIV and 38.4 million people are living with HIV.[17] Women and girls accounted for about 50% of all new infections. In sub-Saharan Africa, women and girls accounted for 63% of all new HIV infections in 2021. Key populations who face increased risk of HIV also often face additional legal and social barriers, including people who use or inject drugs, sex workers and their clients, and LGBTQ+ people.[ii]

In 2022, 274 million people will need humanitarian assistance and protection. This number is a significant increase from 235 million people a year ago, which was already the highest figure in decades.[18] Displaced people and refugees, and especially young people, face increased risks of sexual violence, unwanted pregnancy, sexually transmitted infections (STIs) and unsafe abortion.

Responding to needs

The basis of IPPF advocacy is the recognition of sexual and reproductive rights as basic human rights. It is this position which IPPF, as an NGO, promotes when others too close to national governments may find it difficult to explicitly endorse. Increasingly, IPPF plays a role of convener, building social movements in support of sexual and reproductive rights led by local actors and activists.

By providing an integrated package of essential services through its clinics and outreach programmes, IPPF Member Associations ensure people have access to quality and affordable care that would otherwise not be available through the full life cycle, covering comprehensive sexuality education, contraception, abortion, STIs, including HIV and HPV, infertility, pre- and postnatal care, sexual and gender-based violence, and sexuality counselling.

A key focus for IPPF is to frame sexuality positively, making information and care more responsive to young people's and adolescents' needs. This includes critical areas such as pleasure, enjoyment and diversity that are often left out of discussion due to social and political barriers. With changing gender norms, comprehensive sexuality education should not be limited to education, but should lead to safer options for seeking care so that all young people are equipped with skills to live fulfilling and pleasurable lives and are safe from coercion and violence.

The advances in technology are transforming the way IPPF is delivering care. These adaptations to service delivery models were accelerated during the COVID-19 pandemic. Member Associations had to show exceptional resilience, establishing alternatives to in-clinic care, including digital health, supported self-care and home-based care. For instance, telemedicine and digital platforms have ensured the provision of essential sexual and reproductive healthcare, including abortion, contraception, and sexual and gender-based violence screening and support.[19]

These models of care are an essential and effective part of service delivery, not just during health emergencies, but also for ongoing sustainable care that is focused on client needs and preferences and designed in a way that complements, but does not substitute for, face-to-face care.

The COVID-19 pandemic has spotlighted growing economic and health inequalities, further compounded by the increase in people impacted by climate crisis and conflicts. The ability to respond quickly and effectively to humanitarian crises requires regular adaptations in service delivery models, partnerships and internal processes.[20]

Where next?

IPPF celebrated its 70-year anniversary and launched a new six-year strategy at the end of 2022. This provided an opportunity for the federation to reflect on its history and legacy, including a recognition of the historical and structural power asymmetries that exist between the IPPF Secretariat and Member Associations, but also with international research institutions, funders, international NGOs and UN agencies. These historical power structures reflect the current power structures within the sexual and reproductive health sector, the global health sector and the development aid agenda, and are not unique to IPPF. Identifying mechanisms that place Member Associations at the centre, leveraging the capacities that already exist, and developing a federation across which these can be more effectively acknowledged and shared are priorities now and for the years to come.

My route

My path to public health, and specifically sexual and reproductive health and international development, was not unusual – in the sense that it combined both passion and determination. From my time in secondary school, I had a special interest in history and human geography and developed a real thirst for learning about people's and cultural diversity. This naturally led me to study sociology and social anthropology at Brussels University, where I specifically focused on the impact of culture and values on every aspect of people's lives, including socio-economic order, family relationships, social hierarchy, sexuality and health. While my degree in social anthropology gave me sound qualitative research skills, I decided to complete my education with stronger quantitative competencies and, thanks to a grant from the British Council, I came to England to study medical demography at the London School of Hygiene and Tropical Medicine. I never anticipated that this personal path would lead me to work for an NGO like IPPF.

It would be fair to say that I came to IPPF through chance, although my determination to find a career that would allow me to apply my knowledge and interest in social sciences definitely helped. Following an advertisement in a national newspaper, I successfully applied for a job in the IPPF South Asia Regional Office in 1992. I then joined the London Office in 2001, where I worked in different capacities, including as Senior Abortion Adviser. I came to this role both through my commitment for an issue that is heavily politicised and stigmatised, and thus too often side-lined by other organisations and donors, as well as through the opportunity to lead a large multi-country programme focusing on improving access to abortion care in Africa and South and South East Asia.

My role

I have been working as Director of Global Programmes since 2019. My current task includes overseeing medical and technical capacity sharing, including gender and inclusion and youth. My portfolio also includes overseeing the IPPF humanitarian programme and the procurement of reproductive health supplies. Another key function of my division relates to impact, evidence (including data management and research) and knowledge sharing. The key challenge with such a broad mandate is to keep focused, prioritise and build a strong team of experts able to effectively lead their respective area of work. The ability to identify skills within and outside the organisation, especially looking close to where programmes are implemented, also enables more context-specific and relevant guidance and technical support or accompaniment to be provided to IPPF Member Associations and partners.

This is a challenging role which demands a clear commitment to the organisation's mission and values, strong people and leadership skills, long and irregular working hours, flexibility, diplomacy and sensitivity to different economic and cultural contexts. The competencies required to perform my role include a strong understanding of public health, and specifically sexual and reproductive health and rights, experience working in a wide range of countries especially from the Global South, excellent written and verbal communication skills, and programme management, including budgeting.

Working for an organisation like IPPF is a true privilege. The challenges are many, but they are far outweighed by the rewards and job satisfaction. You can expect long hours and frequent travels, which can take their toll on social and family relationships and make it very difficult to manage a good work/life balance. Thankfully, this is now mitigated by the opportunities offered by technology to work from home when needed.

It also comes with a sense of humility, one that pushes us to question the many assumptions used in our current aid model and challenge the power imbalance it inherently creates. Unlike more centralised international organisations today, the federated structure of IPPF can shift from a model that perpetuates power in a global, often Northern-based, centre to one that releases the power of national actors and civil movements and communities, for programmes that are truly inclusive and person-centred.

Getting started

Students and professionals looking for a career in public health and specifically in international development in an NGO like IPPF do not all need to follow a similar path. They may be doctors, nurses, lawyers, social scientists or others. What they need is a sound technical knowledge in their respective field and strong interpersonal skills. An appreciation of and experience working in the Global South would certainly be a strong asset and so would the knowledge of languages other than English, especially French or Spanish. This can be obtained through professional but also voluntary work or research placement/internships abroad. The road to such a career may be long, and will therefore require patience, tenacity and good networking skills. It also requires flexibility and adaptability, especially in this increasingly challenging political and financial environment. It is important to carefully research opportunities, ask for possible internships, send CVs and contact staff working in fields of particular interest.

Notes

i See Part 4.
ii Lesbian, Gay, Bisexual, Transgender, Questioning and Plus represents other sexual identities.

References

1. Nikendei, C., Cranz, A. and Bugaj, T.J. Medical education and the COVID-19 pandemic – a dress rehearsal for the 'climate pandemic'? *GMS J Med Educ.*, 38(1): Doc. 29, 2021; Goldberg, N. Column: COVID was a dress rehearsal for global climate change. And it didn't go well. *Los Angeles Times*, 9 August 2021. Available at: www.latimes.com/opinion/story/2021-08-09/ipcc-report-covid-climate.
2. King, N.B. and Koski, A. Defining global health as public health somewhere else. *BMJ Global Health*, 5: e002172, 2020.
3. WHO. *Everybody's Business: Strengthening Health Systems to Improve Health Outcomes: WHO's Framework for Action*, 2007. Available at: https://apps.who.int/iris/handle/10665/43918.
4. WHO. Health for All by 2000, 1981. Available at: https://apps.who.int/iris/bitstream/handle/10665/38893/9241800038.pdf?sequence=1; Department of Health. *Health Is Global: An Outcomes Framework for Global Health 2011–2015*, 2011.
5. Department of Health, 2011, op. cit.
6. HM Treasury and Department for International Development. *UK Aid: Tackling Global Challenges in the National Interest*, 23 November 2015. Available at: www.gov.uk/government/publications/uk-aid-tackling-global-challenges-in-the-national-interest.
7. McKinsey & Company. *Ten Innovations that Can Improve Global Health*. Available at: www.mckinsey.com/industries/healthcare-systems-and-services/our-insights/ten-innovations-that-can-improve-global-health.
8. WHO. *World Health Day 2022*. Available at: www.who.int/campaigns/world-health-day/2022.
9. GOV.UK *Guidance: Public Health Skills and Knowledge Framework (PHSKF)*. Available at: www.gov.uk/government/publications/public-health-skills-and-knowledge-framework-phskf.
10. IPPF. *2021 Annual Performance Report*. Available at: www.ippf.org/resource/2021-annual-performance-report.
11. Starrs, A.M. *et al.*, Accelerate Progress – Sexual and Reproductive Health and Rights for All: Report of the Guttmacher-Lancet Commission. *Lancet.* 391(June 30): 2642–89, 2018.
12. IPPF. Humanitarian Strategy 2018–2022. Available at: www.ippf.org/sites/default/files/2018-06/IPPF%20-%20Humanitarian%20Strategy%202018_FINAL.pdf.
13. UN Population Fund. *Minimum Initial Service Package (MISP) for SRH in Crisis Situations*. Available at: www.unfpa.org/resources/minimum-initial-service-package-misp-srh-crisis-situations#:~:text=The%20Minimum%20Initial%20Service%20Package,onset%20of%20a%20humanitarian%20crisis.
14. Lancet Commission. *Sexual and Reproductive Health and Rights for All: Report of the Guttmacher*, 9 May 2018. Available at: www.thelancet.com/journals/lancet/article/PIIS0140-6736(18)30293-9/fulltext.
15. Starrs *et al.*, 2018, op. cit.

16. Reproductive Health Supplies Commission. *Commodity Gap Analysis*. Available at: www.rhsupplies.org/cga/.
17. UN AIDS. *Global HIV & AIDS Statistics – Fact Sheet*. Available at: www.unaids.org/en/resources/fact-sheet.
18. UN Office for the Co-ordination of Humanitarian Affairs. *Global Humanitarian Overview 2022*. Available at: https://2022.gho.unocha.org/.
19. IPPF. *Delivering No Matter What: IPPF's Response to the COVID-19 Pandemic*. Available at: www.ippf.org/resource/delivering-no-matter-what-ippfs-response-covid-19-pandemic.
20. UN Population Fund. *Impact of COVID-19 on Family Planning: What We Know One Year into the Pandemic*. Available at: www.unfpa.org/resources/impact-covid-19-family-planning-what-we-know-one-year-pandemic.

8 Sustainability and climate change

Jenny Griffiths; David Pencheon;
Isobel Braithwaite; Fiona Sim; Jenny Wright

Introduction to this challenge

Climate change is at last recognised as an urgent, major public health – and existential – challenge now facing the world. That is why we are dedicating a whole section of this book to it. Direct involvement of public health professionals in climate change and sustainability as a discrete and specialised area of work is relatively new, although there has been, of course, input for many years, into both research and practice, in improving air quality, transport and planning to mediate the effects of harmful emissions on the health of the population. Indeed, what is increasingly commonly set out as the Green Agenda has very quickly become an underpinning theme, as inequalities have done, to all of public health practice. The public health workforce can use its skills in leadership, advocacy, epidemiology and evidence communication to influence policy makers at all levels.

Challenges and opportunities – vision for public health's contribution to this major issue

Jenny Griffiths, Public Health and Climate Change Activist

The climate and environmental crisis – the ultimate opportunity for all public health practitioners

The United Nations' powerful framework of 17 Sustainable Development Goals[1] – one of which is, of course, climate action – inspires my vision of public health. We need to live and breathe the knowledge that the climate crisis, linked with the precipitous recent decline in the abundance and diversity of the natural world, is the greatest threat to public health (indeed to life itself) this century.

As the Earth's climate system breaks down, the dangers are visibly increasing – long droughts, more frequent severe storms and floods, and record-breaking temperatures during heatwaves. Greenhouse gas emissions (GHGs) must be reduced by two-thirds by 2030 to give us a chance of

DOI: 10.4324/9781003433699-10

keeping global warming below the 'safe' level of 1.5 degrees. If we fail, unstable weather will increasingly damage agriculture and therefore food supply; and growing numbers of people will be displaced from areas of the world rendered uninhabitable by sea-level rise or desertification.

All this is a call to arms for public health, providing us with a driving, unifying purpose, a massive opportunity to improve human health. Every Director of Public Health should see the environment as central to their work and – while there are already some – there should be many more jobs focused on climate action. Indeed, *all* careers – in health protection, health improvement, healthcare public health, public health intelligence and academic public health – afford the opportunity to advocate for rapid action to reduce GHGs. My vision is that leadership and advocacy for tackling the climate crisis features strongly in the role descriptions of all public health jobs.

What is good for the climate is good for health. All of us should model pro-environmental behaviours and demonstrate low-carbon ways of living. We can communicate simple messages in our day-to-day working lives: that a healthy diet is often also a low-carbon diet (that is, little or no red meat), and the health benefits of walking and cycling. We can also promote multifunctional green spaces for physical and mental health, growing local food and improving biodiversity.

Public health practitioners are well placed to link health and social inequalities and climate justice and help those struggling to live sustainably and healthily. For example, as well as reducing carbon emissions, investment in insulation and retrofitting with low-carbon forms of heating using renewable energy help those who cannot afford to heat their homes properly.

We in public health must also assist local communities in adapting to the impacts of the climate crisis, especially if (as seems increasingly likely[2]) global warming rises beyond two degrees. Houses need to be adapted to cope with heatwaves without energy-guzzling air conditioning. We need to grow more of our own food locally, to be more self-sufficient when supplies fail. But there will be rewards. As Sir David Attenborough said in his address to the COP26 Climate Summit on 1 November 2021: 'We will all share in the benefits. Affordable, clean energy, healthy air and enough food to sustain us.'[3]

I am pleased that the Faculty of Public Health has a strong Climate and Health Strategy and environmental sustainability is embedded within the specialty training curriculum. Public health practitioners have vital leadership, advocacy and influencing skills.

I have always believed strongly in multi-disciplinary public health. People from a very wide range of backgrounds, including the voluntary sector and community development, working and learning together is the only way to tackle the complexity of a crisis that the UN Secretary-General has described as 'code red for humanity'.[4]

Overview of public health's contribution to climate change and sustainability

David Pencheon, Honorary Professor, Health and Sustainable Development, Exeter University

Reflections on sustainability and climate change as an important and urgent public health endeavour

What is the place of action on climate change as part of the big health and justice issues of the day? What can and should the public health workforce be doing? What are the implications for training? A new approach is developing quickly.

There is good and ample scientific evidence of the issues that need to be addressed (extreme weather events, migration, global injustice, GHG emissions, poorly resilient and unhealthy food systems ...). Large-scale collective actions globally are needed, with most current actions derived from a value-based endeavour from people who care about it, rather than from rational people, organisations and governments who are too good at denying, disavowing and delaying. Actions from every health professional are needed, both at home and at work. An important barrier to be overcome is the competitiveness of 'my action is more important than yours' – the complete opposite of a collective, large-scale systems approach to addressing the grave challenges and enabling the huge opportunities.

A systems-wide approach

It is important to learn how different perspectives and actions on health and climate change can interact and reinforce the effectiveness of one another to produce multiple benefits in time and place. As professionals learn, we inevitably gravitate to understand some areas in depth, but this should not give us the excuse to ignore the interconnectedness of everything – and a more system-wide, global approach to issues such as poverty, oppression, human rights and climate change. How do we help one another respect all the big issues we are faced with? Public health is a methodological discipline which can be applied widely, but one of the key contributions of the discipline is to frame and quantify the big issues of public health and justice and mediate a path to a safe and secure future.

A sustainable development approach weaves together the social, environmental and economic causes of health, especially over the long term. It cannot be over-focused only on the environment nor the immediate, but has to be part of the social global determinants of health and inequalities, appreciating the social, economic and environmental causes of both health and disease – hence the constant need for a systems approach, in thinking, understanding, engaging and acting.

A new approach for public health

Epidemiology may be the core scientific discipline in public health, but we need to separate out cause and effect and place it in the broad spectrum of systems thinking. Indeed, using only classical epidemiological techniques risks closing minds to the importance of more complex and nuanced approaches to cause and effect, which are fundamental to systems thinking. Most people prefer to study relationships which are concrete, simple and content-focused. The skill in public health is not to be too attached to one methodological approach: we have to appreciate which methods can best be applied in which circumstances. If an individual prefers to work with one methodological approach, then that person needs to work as part of a team and respect the approaches adopted by other people. 'Pure' can mean 'siloed'. This means public health professionals must know their own strengths and have insight – to know if and when they may need to work with others to deliver the best outcomes for all, now and in the future. They need to have both breadth (to appreciate the larger picture and systems) and sufficient depth (where they can apply their own particular expertise as part of a collective endeavour).

When there are large-scale, disruptive, existential threats, it can often be most effective for professionals with a strong moral purpose (for example, health professionals) to be acting both within and from outside the tent. Trainees need to be empowered and supported to take the initiative, to take risks, to be clear, to state if there is uncertainty in the evidence, to speak truth to power. Public health professionals have a rich heritage in listening up, sitting up, standing up, and speaking out about the big issues of health and justice with humility in an engaging and honest way. No one is an absolute expert.

Public health, of course, embraces new areas, but is too often involved too late. A key skill in public health is to talk with humility about uncertainty, with moral authority, and with clear understanding of the most reliable data and research available. This includes a narrative framing of the issues, both problems and solutions, which engage the many value sets that exist, for as many people as possible. Most of us forget that communicating means as much listening as talking. We do not necessarily need to mention the words 'public health' when talking about big health issues such as climate change. We can – and should – talk about the health of the population as a collective endeavour, not as a cadre of officials. We need to be fit for task, not just fit for a 'profession'. The issue at stake with climate change is about the safeguarding of civilisation and the living systems on which it depends. There are many excellent overviews of the state of the planet.[5]

How do seismic system changes happen? Often without anyone noticing at first. One day we are operating from one set of rules, with one set of values. And then suddenly we are doing something else. How did that happen? The art and science of large-scale change does include engagement, science, tactics, vision and strategy as one might expect. But it also includes other skills such as being attentive to where the appetite for change really is at any one time, and creating the conditions such that change is more likely in broadly the right direction (as one never knows exactly what the immediate future opportunities hold). It sometimes involves different sorts of leadership, such as opportunism and flexibility, and it always involves seeking a broad mandate and building on what people are already doing.

Keeping an open mind to trigger points for change

As is so often the case, the future has already arrived; it is just a little unevenly distributed. The NHS has pledged to achieve net zero carbon emissions by 2040. Other countries ask us how we got the government/Department of Health and Social Care to agree to that. People work on micro changes, then suddenly everyone is doing it. The science of social tipping points – be they in tobacco usage or pro-social behaviour – is surely a key public health skill. What do we need to do to move from banging at the door to make the case for change, to suddenly finding the door is wide open; how must one's approach and method of engagement change in such circumstances? What is the tipping point, the trigger? One can never be exactly sure. It is not just mechanical or technical interventions that create that change – it is a profoundly human and often unknowable set of circumstances. One has to be open to every model of change and to be ready to try all approaches, to try all things. What is the trigger now for global climate change action; when do individual actions lead to population movement? The only way is through collective action rather than competitive action. We need to surf uncertain waves, to be able to navigate complexity. Success in any one area will also generally lead to improvement elsewhere in the system.

Finding innovative solutions

In sustainability, like most public health actions, it is not enough simply to exhort, point fingers and attribute blame. We do have to show what needs to be done about it; being practical, personal and possible. Public health has too often been focused on problems rather than on presenting solutions. We must also think in systems, to help ourselves and others think outside our comfort zones, which may seem unnatural and uncomfortable to some. We need to go where it is difficult, and walk towards the problems.

Climate collapse is happening on our watch and how we react and cope and build a foundation for a better future will be our legacy.

Career story

Isobel Braithwaite, National Institute for Health and Care Research
Academic Clinical Fellow in Public Health, University College London

How I started on a public health career

I went to medical school with thoughts of one day working as a doctor for a humanitarian or development charity – I think this is because I had a strong conviction that everyone should have access to the healthcare and other essentials that they needed, irrespective of where they lived, and I wanted to help make that a reality. I liked science and spending time with people, so medicine seemed a natural fit. However, my knowledge of both global and public health at that time was limited, and these 'bigger picture' subjects featured little in my undergraduate teaching. Particularly in the earlier years, this focused largely on the intricacies of human anatomy and on the cellular and molecular processes that keep us alive or cause disease, but very little on why the diseases we studied were often much more common in deprived areas and groups, or the causes of the stark differences in health outcomes between richer and poorer parts of the world.

Having signed up to the mailing list of a student-led global health organisation, then Medsin (now Students for Global Health), as a first-year medical student, an email dropped into my inbox one day. It offered the chance to attend a training programme about the links between climate change, health and the NHS, which would be focused on giving participants knowledge and skills to drive changes at a local level. Something that I found I kept returning to after the weekend-long crash course was a slide that showed graphically the clear and unjust contrast between the countries most responsible for climate change and who was already paying the price with their lives (Figure 8.1).

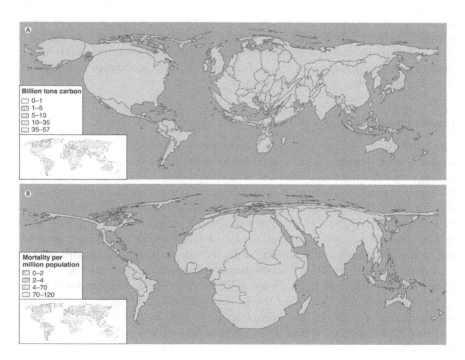

Figure 8.1 Comparison of undepleted cumulative CO_2 emissions by country for 1950–2000 versus the regional distribution of four climate-sensitive health consequences (malaria, malnutrition, diarrhoea and inland flood-related fatalities) (Costello *et al.*, 2009[6])

Images reproduced with permission from *The Lancet*.

The image in Figure 8.1 is from the first UCL-Lancet Commission on Climate Change and Health, and while the numbers have changed in the intervening years, the broad pattern has not. It may sound clichéd, but what I learned from that programme and the people I met as a result led to a major change in how I saw climate change. I came to recognise it as intimately connected with both global and more local causes of ill health, and as a real and present danger that was far less under control than I had assumed.

As I learned more about the impacts of rising temperatures, sea-level rise and extreme weather on both physical and mental health, I grew increasingly alarmed by the major threat I could see that climate change posed to both health and health equity, and was perplexed and worried by how little it featured in my medical training. As a result, most of the students around me still had no awareness of the risks I had started to learn about and become more conscious of.

My reading and thinking around this also turned my latent interest in the large-scale societal forces that influence health into something more active. In terms of my career plans, I felt increasingly sure that I wanted my work to focus more on prevention than treatment, and that led to my interest in career options in public health. At the same time, I also felt a need to try to connect that to addressing climate change and its causes, because of the ways in which climate and environmental breakdown tend to multiply and exacerbate so many existing social issues, from poverty and inequality to homelessness, migration and potentially conflict.

Courses and qualifications

Over the course of my time at medical school, I sought out opportunities to learn more about these areas and to contribute, becoming involved in a range of organisations, projects and campaigns. I volunteered and did a summer internship with the Centre for Sustainable Healthcare, working to develop their SHE (sustainable healthcare education) network, and was part of a team which published a set of sustainable healthcare learning outcomes in *The Lancet*. Around that time, I realised that I wanted a stronger grounding in the principles and technical skills that underpin public health science and practice, and in 2013 I was fortunate in being able to take a year out of my medical training to study for a Master's in Public Health, specialising in Environment and Health, at the London School of Hygiene and Tropical Medicine, before returning to complete the second half of medical school.

From that point onwards, I became increasingly involved in grassroots organising and advocacy alongside my studies, taking on the role of national coordinator for the student group Healthy Planet UK, organising peer-to-peer training for other students, and building an advocacy coalition campaigning for health institutions such as the British Medical Association, Wellcome Trust and various Royal Colleges to move all of their investments (divest) away from fossil fuels. Later on, I started volunteering and then working part time for the Global Climate and Health Alliance, helping to organise international conferences on climate change and health at two COP climate summits,[i] coordinating advocacy declarations and reports, and bringing new organisations into the Alliance.

Public health posts held

After finishing my medical training, I spent a couple of years working in London hospitals as a junior doctor. I managed to organise a taster week based with a nearby local authority's public health team during my first year as a Foundation trainee doctor, and was fascinated by the breadth of different activities and issues they dealt with, and their ways of working with the local community. The following year, I had a four-month-long rotation in mental health research, which I spent working on a project investigating the relationship between air pollution and mental health. My involvement in climate and sustainability work before then had shown me that air pollution, including some of the substances most harmful to health such as particulate matter and nitrogen dioxide, is an important part of the climate-health challenge, both because of its direct health impacts and because these pollutants are often produced alongside various GHGs, and so reducing air pollution offers many 'co-benefits' for health and climate. I led a systematic review of the literature to explore whether air pollution affected mental health, as was already well-established for many physical health conditions, and found a range of studies which together suggested an adverse impact of long-term air pollution (particulate matter) exposure on depression risk.

Working as a Foundation trainee doctor was often both emotionally and physically demanding, and – outside of my academic rotation – I found it difficult to stay as actively involved in work related to climate, sustainability and health as I would have liked to during those two years. I loved the patient contact and teamwork that the role demanded, but at the same time was frustrated at many of the hospital systems and how little I was able to do to address the root causes of many of my patients' illnesses, from social isolation and poverty, to the unhealthy homes and environments they lived in.

Those two years helped confirm my sense that I might be better suited to working in public health and tackling health problems further 'upstream'. I also felt that specialising in public health was likely to open up more opportunities for me to contribute to climate change mitigation and adaptation within my work. So I applied to join the public health specialty training scheme and was offered a training post in London, spending my first year as a public health registrar at Camden and Islington local authorities from mid-2018. I worked on several projects, ranging from reducing smoking in pregnancy and improving uptake of cervical screening among under-served community groups, to a Needs Assessment on self-harm in children and young people across the two boroughs, and a shorter report on air pollution in Camden. I also took the Faculty of Public Health's Part A (Diplomate) Exam that year, which refreshed key concepts and methods from my Master's and has provided a strong foundation for my subsequent work.

Since then, I have been able to experience many different sides of public health through different registrar placements (as part of the higher specialist training scheme[ii]), both before and – primarily – during the COVID-19 pandemic. This has included working in response to a range of infectious disease outbreaks, incidents and enquiries with the North East and Central London Health Protection Team in late 2019, and then with the Extreme Events team in Public Health England (now UKHSA), which I sought out because of my interest in climate and health. I joined the Extreme Events team from January to September 2020, responding to storms and floods and – once the pandemic hit – working on a framework to help decision-makers at local level address intersecting risks from heatwaves and COVID-19. Through an Academic Clinical Fellowship, I had opportunities to undertake various research projects at University College London's Institute for Health Informatics, including work looking at the unequal impacts of COVID-19 in UK prisons and homeless populations and working on the UCL Virus Watch study led by Professors Rob Aldridge and Andrew Hayward.

In spring 2021, I joined the Greater London Authority's Health Team, which involved a range of reactive work and briefings related to COVID-19 alongside longer-term work. The latter included bringing key health partners together with a focus on improving air quality in London, feeding into regional and local plans around pandemic recovery, and on work to scale up an ambitious programme ('School Superzones') aiming to create healthier areas around London's schools, through locally designed changes.[7]

Over the course of 2020–2021, I applied for a National Institute for Health Research Doctoral Fellowship, in order to undertake a PhD at UCL focusing on the health impacts of cold and energy-inefficient housing, which I was awarded and began in May 2022 (having applied for an 'OOPR' or 'Out of Programme for Research' period of three years, so that I can return to complete my public health training at the end of the PhD). During the Fellowship, I am reviewing the state of the current evidence base regarding long-term health risks of living in energy-inefficient and cold housing, and the health benefits of energy-efficiency improvements, and aiming to establish and make use of two new data linkages between health and housing (energy performance) data, in order to improve our understanding of the burden of disease and to inform policy in this area.

The challenges and rewards of my role

On first starting public health training, it took me some time to adjust to the much more long-term nature of local authority public health work after the fast pace of being a junior doctor, and the much less frequent interaction with patients and their families. At the same time, I enjoyed the work and felt that it had been the right career move for me. I love having the chance to get to grips with a wide range of complex and interconnected social and health challenges and to work in partnership with many different people, each bringing their own skills and perspectives, to try and steer some of these seemingly intractable issues in a better direction. I also really value the emphasis of the public health specialty training programme on continual learning and development – including the ability to go out of programme and do research for an extended period, such as for a PhD, and the huge variety of topics and skills this can cover.

During the COVID-19 pandemic, the public health workforce has faced many challenges, from often heavy workloads, keeping abreast of rapidly changing evidence and guidance and needing to make decisions despite uncertainty, as well as the dissolution of Public Health England and its replacement by the UKHSA and the Office for Health Improvement and Disparities (OHID), all during 2021. At the same time, I have learned so much over this period, and feel lucky to have had so many passionate, thoughtful and supportive colleagues. For me, often the people you get to work with are definitely one of the best parts of a career in public health.

Maintaining a work/life balance

I've become more aware over time that there is always more that can be done in both public health and in relation to the climate crisis, irrespective of how long or hard you work, which risks exhaustion and burnout, particularly if you try to shoulder too much on your own. I think this is partly why I have sought out a career that gives me significant scope to set my own direction and enables me to spend more of my working hours trying to tackle the issues that I care most about, rather than staying in clinical work and burning the candle at both ends with climate- and health-related organising and activism alongside full-time work commitments.

Over time, I have learned how important 'personal sustainability' is, alongside how sustainability is usually understood. I try to leave more space outside of work for what sustains me – like time with the people closest to me, getting outdoors, exercise, good food, rest – and to accept the limits on what I can do. I'm sure I'll need to keep working on that balance throughout my career and as I take on new challenges, but I've been really glad to see the beginnings of a more open conversation around work/life balance and related issues like gender and disability equality in many public health organisations over the past few years.

Notes

i Conference of the Parties (COP) is a series spanning three decades of UN Climate Change Conferences.
ii See Part 4.

References

1. United Nations. *The 17 Goals*. Available at: https://sdgs.un.org/goals.
2. UN *Emissions Gap Report 2022* published ahead of COP27 in October 2022. Available at: https://www.unep.org/resources/emissions-gap-report-2022.
3. David Attenborough COP26 Climate Summit Glasgow Speech Transcript. Available at: https://www.rev.com/blog/transcripts/david-attenborough-cop26-climate-summit-glasgow-speech-transcript.
4. UN Secretary-General, Antonio Guterres, in his address to the General Assembly as the UN Headquarters in New York, 26 October 2021.
5. Wallace-Wells, D. *The Uninhabitable Earth*, London, Allen Lane, 1st edn, 2019.
6. Costello, A., Abbas, M., Allen, A., Ball, B., Bell, S. and Bellamy, R. Managing the health effects of climate change. *The Lancet*, 373(9676), 2009.
7. Mayor of London. *School Superzones*. Available at: https://www.london.gov.uk/what-we-do/health/school-superzones.

Public health functions – useful resources

Health improvement

Local Government Association. *Public Health and Prevention*. Available at: www.local.gov.uk/our-support/our-improvement-offer/care-and-health-improvement/public.

NHS Race & Health Observatory. *Ethnic Inequalities in Healthcare: A Rapid Evidence Review*. Available at: www.nhsrho.org/wp-content/uploads/2022/02/RHO-Rapid-Review-Final-Report_Summary_v.4.pdf.

Northern Health Science Alliance. *Child of the North: Building a Fairer Future after COVID-19*. Available at: www.thenhsa.co.uk/app/uploads/2022/01/Child-of-the-North-Report-FINAL-1.pdf.

Sheffield DPH. *Left Shift. Show Me the Evidence*. Available at: https://gregfellpublichealth.wordpress.com/2021/11/18/left-shift-show-me-the-evidence/.

University of Cambridge. *Levelling Up Health: A Practical, Evidence-Based Framework*. Available at: www.phpc.cam.ac.uk/pcu/research/research-groups/crmh/research/crmh-health-inequalities/levelling-up-health-a-practical-evidence-based-framework/.

Health intelligence

Institute for Apprenticeships & Technical Education. *Health and Care Intelligence Specialist*. Available at: www.instituteforapprenticeships.org/apprenticeship-standards/health-and-care-intelligence-specialist-v1-0.

Careers guidance:

NHS. *Public Health Knowledge and Intelligence Professional*. Available at: www.healthcareers.nhs.uk/explore-roles/public-health/roles-public-health/public-health-knowledge-and-intelligence-professional.

Free course:

NHS England. *elearning for healthcare*. Available at: www.e-lfh.org.uk.

DOI: 10.4324/9781003433699-11

Professional accreditation:

Association of Professional Healthcare Analysts website. Available at: www.aph analysts.org.
Federation for Informatics Professionals website. Available at: www.fedip.org.

State of the profession:

Centre for Workforce Intelligence. *The Public Health Knowledge and Intelligence Workforce: A CfWI Study.* Available at: chrome-extension://efaidnbmnnnibpcajp cglclefindmkaj/https://assets.publishing.service.gov.uk/government/uploads/system/ uploads/attachment_data/file/507593/CfWI_PH_Knowledge_and_Intelligence_ Workforce.pdf.

Healthcare public health

Help with research opportunities

The NIHR Nursing & Midwifery Incubator in partnership with the Research Design Service has created a virtual advisory service to help aspiring clinical academic midwives to advance their research careers:
Clinical Academic Career Advisory Service.
National Institute for Health and Care Research. *NIHR Fellowship Programme.* Available at: www.nihr.ac.uk/explore-nihr/academy-programmes/fellowship-programme. htm.

Funding support for research

The Iolanthe Midwifery Trust provides grants to midwives. The website is available at: www.iolanthe.org/.
The Nightingale Fund provides support towards fees for post-qualification education to nurses, midwives and public health nurses. The website is available at: www. thenightingalefund.uk/.
Royal College of Nursing. *Scholarships and Bursaries.* Available at: www.rcn.org.uk/ professional-development/scholarships-and-bursaries/mary-seacole-awards.

Health protection

The function of health protection

European Commission. *The EU–UK Trade and Cooperation Agreement.* Available at: https://commission.europa.eu/strategy-and-policy/relations-non-eu-countries/ relations-united-kingdom/eu-uk-trade-and-cooperation-agreement_en.
Faculty of Public Health. *Functions and Standards of a Public Health System.* Available at: chrome-extension://efaidnbmnnnibpcajpcglclefindmkaj/https://www.fph.org. uk/media/3031/fph_systems_and_function-final-v2.pdf.
Health Protection Policy Toolkit: Health as an Essential Component of Global Security, Commonwealth Secretariat/Public Health Wales. Available at: www.the commonwealth.io/wp-content/uploads/2020/05/Health-Protection-Policy-Toolkit. pdf.

The Health Security (EU Exit) Regulations 2021. Available at: www.legislation.gov.
uk/ukdsi/2021/9780348224375/introduction.

World Health Organization. *International Health Regulations*. Available at: www.
who.int/health-topics/international-health-regulations#tab=tab_1.

World Health Organization Regional Office for Europe. *The 10 Essential Public Health
Operations*. Available at: www.euro.who.int/en/health-topics/Health-systems/
public-health-services/policy/the-10-essential-public-health-operations.

Dealing with pandemics and incidents

CDC. *Importance of One Health for Covid-19 and Future Pandemics*. Available at:
www.cdc.gov/media/releases/2021/s1103-one-health.html.

UK Parliament. *The Salisbury Incident: Research Briefing*, House of Commons
Library. Available at: https://commonslibrary.parliament.uk/research-briefings/cdp-
2018-0204/.

GOV.UK. Radiation Incidents: Public Health Preparedness and Response. Available at: www.gov.uk/government/collections/radiation-incidents-public-health-
preparedness-and-response.

The King's Fund. *Directors of Public Health and the Covid-19 Pandemic: 'A Year
Like No Other'*. Available at: www.kingsfund.org.uk/publications/directors-public-
health-covid-19-pandemic.

OECD. *Environmental Health and Strengthening Resilience to Pandemics*. Available at: www.oecd.org/coronavirus/policy-responses/environmental-health-and-
strengthening-resilience-to-pandemics-73784e04/.

World Health Organization. *A Year without Precedent: WHO's Covid-19 Response*, December 2020. Available at: https://who.int/news-room/spotlight/a-year-
without-precedent-who-s-covid-19-response.

World Health Organization. *Communicable Disease Surveillance and Response
System: Guide to Monitoring and Evaluating*. Available at: chrome-extension://
efaidnbmnnnibpcajpcglclefindmkaj/https://apps.who.int/iris/bitstream/handle/
10665/69331/WHO_CDS_EPR_LYO_2006_2_eng.pdf?sequence=1&isAllowed=y.

Careers in health protection

Chartered Institute of Environmental Health. Available at: www.cieh.org/what-is-
environmental-health/how-do-i-become-an-ehp/.

Chartered Institute of Environmental Health. *Research Shows Environmental Health
Is One of the Best Career Options in a Post-COVID World (England)*. Available
at: www.cieh.org/news/press-releases/2020/research-shows-environmental-health-
is-one-of-the-best-career-options-in-a-post-covid-world-england/.

European Centre for Disease Prevention and Control. *Fellowship Programme: EPIET/
EUPHEM*. Available at: www.ecdc.europa.eu/en/epiet-euphem.

Faculty of Public Health. Health protection and communicable diseases. In: *Health
Knowledge Public Health Textbook*. Available at: www.healthknowledge.org.uk/
public-health-textbook/disease-causation-diagnostic/2g-communicable-disease.

GOV.UK. *Guidance: Apprenticeships that Support Public Health Careers: 2021 Status Update*. Available at: https://gov.uk/government/publications/apprenticeships-
that-support-public-health-careers/apprenticeships-that-support-public-health-
careers-2021-status-update--2.

GOV.UK. Independent Report: *An Overview of Modernising Scientific Careers*. Available at: www.gov.uk/government/publications/an-overview-of-modernising-scientific-careers.

GOV.UK. *UK Field Epidemiology Training Programme (UKFETP)*. Available at: www.gov.uk/guidance/field-epidemiology-training-programme-fetp.

Hawker, J. *Communicable Disease Control and Health Protection Handbook*, 4th edition, Oxford, Wiley, 2019.

NHS. *Public Health Nurse*. Available at: www.healthcareers.nhs.uk/explore-roles/public-health/roles-public-health/public-health-nurse#Health%20protection%20nurse.

NHS. *Roles in Public Health*. Available at: www.healthcareers.nhs.uk/explore-roles/public-health/roles-public-health.

Royal College of Nursing. *Become a Nurse*. Available at: www.rcn.org.uk/professional-development/become-a-nurse.

Royal College of Nursing. *The Value and Contribution of Nursing to Public Health in the UK*. Available at: www.rcn.org.uk/Professional-Development/publications/pub-005497.

TURAS. *Career Development Framework for Health Protection Nursing*. Available at: https://learn.nes.nhs.scot/36216/career-development-framework-for-health-protection-nursing.

Academic public health

Faculty of Public Health. *Academic Public Health Special Interest Group*. Available at: www.fph.org.uk/policy-advocacy/special-interest-groups/special-interest-groups-list/academic-public-health-special-interest-group/.

NHS. *Modernising Medical Careers: Report of the Academic Careers Sub-Committee Modernising Medical Careers and the UK Clinical Research Collaboration* (Walport Report), March 2005. Available at: www.ukcrc.org/wp-content/uploads/2014/03/Medically_and_Dentally-qualified_Academic_Staff_Report.pdf.

Climate change

Committee on Climate Change. *The Sixth Carbon Budget: The UK's Path to Net Zero*. Available at: www.theccc.org.uk/wp-content/uploads/2020/12/The-Sixth-Carbon-Budget-The-UKs-path-to-Net-Zero.pdf.

Faculty of Public Health. *Climate and Health Strategy 2021–25*. Available at: www.fph.org.uk/media/3401/fph-climate-health-strategy-final.pdf.

Faculty of Public Health. *Resources on Climate Change and Health*. Available at: www.fph.org.uk/policy-advocacy/special-interest-groups/special-interest-groups-list/sustainable-development-special-interest-group/resources-on-sustainable-development-and-climate-change/.

Intergovernmental Panel on Climate Change (IPCC). *Climate Change 2021: The Physical Science Basis – Summary for Policymakers*. Available at: www.ipcc.ch/report/ar6/wg1/downloads/report/IPCC_AR6_WGI_SPM_final.pdf.

The Lancet. *The* Lancet *Countdown on Health and Climate Change*. Published annually. Available at: www.thelancet.com/countdown-health-climate.

Part 3

Settings for public health practice

Fiona Sim and Jenny Wright

Introduction

This section looks at three different settings or places in which public health professionals are usually to be found and their presence critical. For each setting, contributors set out why it is such a valuable location from which to work in terms of health and inequality issues, what difference the public health workforce can make, and how to train and acquire practical experience in this setting. The personal career stories demonstrate this in practice.

The three settings highlighted in Part 3 are:

- local government;
- health policy and system leadership; and
- the UK voluntary and community sector.

DOI: 10.4324/9781003433699-12

9 Local government

Sarah Price; Greg Fell; Shakiba Habibula; Fiona Sim; Jenny Wright

Introduction to this setting

Local councils, or local authorities as they are also called, are led by councillors who are elected by local people. Advised by paid officials, councillors make major decisions on the services each council provides, oversee how these services are run and represent the interests of people in the division or ward area they represent. Councillors are normally elected every four years. This element of democracy is key, ensuring public accountability and scrutiny, and distinguishes councils from other public bodies such as the NHS.

Local authorities have a wide range of powers and duties. These vary depending on the type of local authority. County councils have different duties from district or town or parish councils, while unitary authorities, as their name implies, carry all the functions. A number of council collaboratives are classed as Mayoral Combined Authorities. National policy is set by central government, but local councils are responsible for all day-to-day services and local matters. They are mainly funded by the government's revenue support grant, council tax paid by local residents and redistributed business rates. The responsibilities of councils are wide, including a range of functions that can exert influence over health and inequality issues: exactly where public health professionals want to be working to ensure that influence is used to improve the health of local people and to protect them from harm. In England, upper-tier local authorities (unitaries and county councils) are funded to commission or deliver some public health functions. Other responsibilities of councils include:

- education;
- environment, including parks and green spaces;
- housing;
- leisure;
- environmental health, including food safety;
- trading standards;
- local road networks and public transport;
- planning;

DOI: 10.4324/9781003433699-13

- social care;
- community safety; and
- economic development.

The public health workforce in all four UK countries works closely with local government and, in England, local public health teams are directly employed by upper-tier and unitary councils.

The pandemic, as will be evident from the contributions that follow, has had a profound effect on how the public health workforce in local councils is perceived and valued. This now needs to be sustained and built on for the future.

Challenges and opportunities – vision for public health in local government

Sarah Price, Chief for Population Health and Inequalities and Deputy Chief Executive, NHS Greater Manchester Integrated Care

I work for NHS Greater Manchester Integrated Care, part of the Greater Manchester Integrated Care Partnership. It covers a city region that suffers from poorer health than the England average. Smoking, for example, remains a very big public health issue. The Partnership comprises local NHS organisations and local authorities that serve the 2.8 million people who live in Greater Manchester. This builds on the arrangements that came into being in 2016 with the devolution of health and care, with organisations aiming to work as a system to improve health and promote healthy lives. From a public health perspective, it was this that enabled the dedicated partnership team to work with the ten local Directors of Public Health (DsPH) and Public Health England across Greater Manchester, to bring together local and more specialist public health skills to take on a broader 'health determinants' agenda.[i] The Partnership, for example, enabled local neighbourhoods, sports and leisure sectors to work together on improving the levels of physical activity among local people. Working together has proved particularly important given most local authority public health teams are relatively small. Further, many DsPH do not report directly to chief executives in their councils and so their voice may not always be heard when important decisions are made. The Partnership helped support local DsPH, and together exert greater influence on health matters. But I recognise that our model is not typical of the country as a whole.

Greater Manchester was well placed, therefore, to tackle the COVID-19 pandemic on a system-wide basis, getting key population health messages over more consistently. There is no question that the profile of public health has been considerably raised during the pandemic. We must now capitalise on that to make public health more robust within councils with the national funding to support their important work. Local authorities' respect for the skills of DsPH and their teams and their ability to manage emergencies has unquestionably increased: in particular, leading the way in advising the system on testing and contact tracing, visiting safely in care homes and more recently developing a risk framework with Directors of Adult Social Services, allowing admissions to care homes closed due to outbreaks, in a safe and considered way. Enabling a consistent approach across Greater Manchester, without overriding local arrangements, has also been really positive. The pandemic did mean, however, that the focus of public health teams of necessity was on health protection, to the detriment of both health improvement programmes, such as the further roll-out of our CURE programme[1] supporting people to stop smoking when admitted to hospital, as well as of specific initiatives around work and health and service redesign through a healthcare public health lens. I'm optimistic that these programmes will pick up again post-pandemic.

Working with local government can bring enormous benefits. When I worked in Islington as a DPH, a joint appointment between the NHS Primary Care Trust at the time and the local council, we undertook a huge piece of work that matched people with long-term conditions to their housing type and deprivation, in order to target health improvement initiatives to specific groups. Now, with improvements in data processing as well as joint working, we can use data to really influence how we design support for our populations, linking anonymised health experiences alongside other civic data, giving us a much more nuanced approach. I was impressed years ago by the opportunities presented for forming new professional and organisational relationships, and the opportunities to work closely with environmental health, planning and housing, all for the benefit of the health of the local population in a way that was not possible before; an early success was to make the football stadia smoke-free. We must now use the experience from the pandemic to cement our influence within local councils and across communities to accelerate improvement.

Looking to the future, local government is the 'place' leader. Its geography and remit mean it has the ability to reach every area of people's lives and experience. Public health must remain at the heart of local government decision-making, including joint planning,[ii] where it can influence in a way that being located in the NHS cannot always do, although public health should never lose the benefits of being linked to the NHS. We need to strive for the best of both worlds.

Overview of local government as a public health setting

Greg Fell, Director of Public Health, Sheffield City Council

Introduction

Local government is responsible for a very wide range of services for people and businesses in defined areas. Among them are well-known functions such as social care, schools, housing and spatial planning and waste collection, but also lesser-known functions such as leisure, green space, transport and air quality, licensing, environmental health, trading standards, economic strategy, business support, birth and death registrar services, and pest control. Collectively, the contribution these services make to the health of a population is significant.

Local government is organised in different ways across any given geography from unitary council, district council and county council through to Mayoral Combined Authority. The inception of public health in local government started with the role of Medical Officer for Health in the mid-1800s. In 2022, the organisational hosts of much of the public health function are local authorities in England and the NHS in other parts of the UK.

The public health challenges

Gaps between the best and worst geographical areas in life and healthy life expectancy, as well as a significant slowing of the rate of improvement for many indicators, are nothing new. They were well documented in the Marmot Review of 2010.[2] In my area in South Yorkshire, for example, a man living in Dore can expect to live longer than a man living in Darnall, with a seventh of the Dore man's life spent in poor health as opposed to a third in the case of the man in Darnall. Much of that illness and early death is attributable to chronic diseases that are almost entirely preventable. This is a social justice issue as well as an economic issue. There is plenty of evidence that ill health is a significant constraint to economic growth and productivity. Consider the impact of someone who has a heart attack aged 50 and who may not be able to go back to work. This has an impact on the person, their family and, aggregated to a whole population, the economy more broadly.

These issues remain – in fact COVID-19 has exacerbated them. Besides direct impacts on health, the pandemic has had a number of indirect impacts as a result of behaviour change, shifts in patterns of access to services and the effects of lockdowns. This is in addition to the social and economic impacts that will arise downstream. In short, the health of the public is not as good as it could be.

My public health team's time throughout the pandemic has been taken up with organising the response to COVID-19. This has inevitably led to a change in priorities and a shifting of emphasis. In many cases, whole areas of work were left behind. The priority now is to deal with the hidden impacts of the pandemic and take up again those areas which were neglected while refreshing the council's health and wellbeing strategy.

The benefits of cross-department working in reducing inequalities and improving health status

As a team, we are being very mindful of the impact of the pandemic as we reframe the public health service. These are not problems that will be fixed only by better or more health and social care services. A wider approach is needed. Everything a council does contributes to our health and health outcomes, positively or negatively, and this should not be underestimated. Poor quality housing, how we transport ourselves, poverty: all have a huge impact on how healthy we are. Health is as much to do with transport or economic policy or housing policy as it is to do with how much we smoke, or what the NHS and social care do.

In England, public health teams in local government have a budget specifically for public health. It is used to fund services including (but not limited to) health visiting, school nursing, sexual health, drug and alcohol treatment, tobacco control, weight management and obesity, Citizens Advice Bureau, a wide range of community wellbeing services delivered in the voluntary sector and many more. In Sheffield, our service plan is organised around:

- assuring the conditions in which people can live well and be healthy;
- leading with intelligence;
- education, health and care;
- enabling communities; and
- improving the wider determinants of health; protecting health.

Public health roles

Public health in local government and the role of the DPH are not new. They have been around in one form or another for well over 100 years, starting with the Medical Officer of Health at the end of the Victorian era. Public health's historic endeavours have led to enormous advances in the control of communicable disease through immunisation, clean water and sanitation. Some of these issues are still around and, in addition, we have the new health challenges. The public health role has evolved and will continue to evolve over the next 100 years as we act and respond.

Particularly since COVID-19, there has been much emphasis on the role of the DPH. Ours is, however, a team effort. There are some things only public health professionals will own and implement, some where they coordinate and/or lead, some where they provide expert advice and some where they contribute to the agendas of others. Most 'public health', therefore, is done by people who do not have those words in their job title. Poor quality housing, for example, which has a significant bearing on health, is not an issue that public health professionals can solve alone. They have, therefore, to work with and fit multiple frameworks, multiple teams in local government.

A DPH has multiple accountabilities. They may be managerially accountable to the Chief Executive, but will also have links to Regional Directors, the Chief Medical Officer and, within the council, Cabinet Members. The DPH has professional and managerial accountability for all staff in the public health team who need to work across the organisation as they act strategically to shape, influence and support.

Skills needed in the public health workforce

In local government, all of the main areas of public health expertise play their part in how we contribute:

- *Leadership for health* – advocacy, setting a mission and purpose, taking a whole population perspective, translation and interpreting across many different policy areas, understanding of a population's health issues, being highly expert in the scientific aspects of public health – epidemiology, health economics, evidence-based medicine and evaluation.
- *Health improvement* – working with partners on a diverse range of social, economic and environmental issues to ensure the council area is one which supports wellbeing and health for all; tackling smoking, poor diet, alcohol misuse and poor physical activity.
- *Health protection* – intervention and services to improve air quality, water and food, infectious disease control, protection against environmental health hazards, chemical incidents and emergency response.
- *Health intelligence* – surveillance, monitoring and assessment of health and the determinants of health, plus the development of the public health evidence base and knowledge, including the use of behavioural approaches, science and insight. We use our skills in epidemiology and demography to pose questions and provide information. What does the population look like, how will it change, what are the main causes of illness and death, what are the causes of the causes? How is that distributed across a population and how might that change? What are the implications of all that for how a council responds?
- *Support to the NHS and social care* – working with commissioners and providers to ensure that services are accessible, effective, equitable and value for money.

Starting public health careers

The routes into public health in local government are varied. Given the nature of what contributes to 'health', it is easy to see that almost all roles undertaken within local government contribute to the health of the public in some ways. Routes into the profession known as 'public health' can come from any of the wide range of professions that work in local government and beyond. Many departments run apprenticeship schemes that give entry-level opportunities; some will operate informal volunteering opportunities and many will want to work with other organisations and professions in partnership that will give some insight into the day-to-day roles undertaken by public health professionals.[iii]

Public health achievements

There have been improvements in health and the trajectory on many critical indicators of population health is positive. This includes, but is in no way limited to: smoking prevalence, physical activity rates, vaccination rates, cardiovascular mortality, cancer mortality and infant mortality. All of these have not happened by magic, but because many people have done the right things over a sustained period of time.

Why local government provides a rewarding career

Public health is crucial in reducing health inequalities and influencing the wider determinants of health. Local government is, therefore, an important setting for public health work.

Career story

Shakiba Habibula, Consultant in Public Health, Oxfordshire County Council

How I started my career in public health

My involvement in public health was totally unexpected and unplanned! How can you plan when you live in a war zone, when your only concern is your safety and staying alive? Thinking about how I got involved in public health and how it eventually changed my life, I can only think it must have been fate.

I trained as a paediatrician in Afghanistan and my life in public health began before I even knew what it was. I was a young doctor displaced in war-torn Afghanistan from my home in the capital Kabul to the Northern province of Mazar, where I worked for Oxfam and later the UN Children's Fund (UNICEF) looking after people in refugee camps and trying to promote women's and children's health through delivering health education and women's development programmes. This was where I was caught by the magical spell of public health – in an unlikely mix of latrines and the human rights of women.

What brought me to public health

Desperation! War and displacement!

In 1993, in the midst of the civil war in Afghanistan, when I was a young and inexperienced displaced doctor in Mazar province, I needed to find a job in order to survive and feed my family. The one tiny hospital in the city could only offer me an unpaid voluntary job. I searched for jobs high and low until I came across Oxfam. Due to the war in Kabul, most international non-governmental organisations had fled from Kabul and set up offices in the North, which was relatively safe. My medical background was helpful and I got a job with Oxfam supporting its health education and water and sanitation programme for refugees in Mazar. That is where I experienced the magic of public health first-hand. I could see how a simple health education programme could prevent babies from dying unnecessary and avoidable deaths. I could see how educating and up-skilling women could change their status in their families and in the society in which they lived and how all of this impacted on their overall health and wellbeing. I saw how my own life was transformed as a result of my involvement in public health. I had taken a sip from the cup of public health and I wanted to drink deeply.

Relevant training and qualifications

When I started my journey in public health, apart from my medical degree, I had no formal qualification or relevant experience in public health. From my medical training time, all I remembered was a subject called preventive medicine, which was the students' least favourite subject because we thought it was irrelevant to doctors. In our view, we were supposed to learn about how to treat sickness, and preventing disease was someone else's job. Little did I know that public health was more than preventing disease and death, but a social and political movement for bringing about social justice and tackling disparities in society, which are the foundations for achieving good health. I experienced that, first-hand, not only in my own personal life, but in the lives of the thousands of people I worked with in those camps and in the remote villages of Afghanistan.

While working for Oxfam and UNICEF, I felt like I had entered an ocean of public health knowledge without knowing how to swim or navigate my way. I learned, whatever I could, from my boss, a wonderful mentor and coach, but I lacked a solid foundation. It didn't take me long to decide I needed to understand this fascinating field more. Encouraged by my boss, I took the massive step of applying for a Master's Degree in Public Health in Developing Countries at the London School of Hygiene and Tropical Medicine (LSHTM) and that brought me to the UK and started my career path in public health in England.

After obtaining my degree, I was offered a public health research job at the LSHTM by the Health Policy Unit. My boss was a consultant in public health who showed me the ropes and, on his advice, I joined the public health training scheme in Oxford and eventually completed training and secured my first consultant job in 2007. I have never stopped learning and so, to date, I have sought out additional training, including in leadership, teaching, coaching and mentoring, and communication skills.

Posts held

Public health is one of those fields that you can't draw a boundary around. It really is as deep as the ocean and as wide as the sky! I've been very fortunate to have experienced many aspects of this amazing specialty. During my specialist training in public health in the UK, I went through the most exciting training rotation: starting from Berkshire Health Protection Unit, learning the science of preventing infectious diseases; then to Slough Primary Care Trust (PCT), trying to understand the mental health needs of children and young people; I was then attached to Oxfordshire County Council, where I led on a political process negotiating investment in public health priorities through a process called the Local Area Agreement (LAA); then to South East Public Health Observatory, taking part in developing local health profiles in order to bring the health needs of our population to the attention of policy makers; then to the English Department of Health, leading on developing a new national policy on preventing childhood obesity; and finally to Oxfordshire PCT, leading on Emergency Planning and Health Protection; before I secured my first consultant job at Milton Keynes PCT.

In Milton Keynes, I led on Practice Based Commissioning (PBC) and commissioning services for cardio-vascular diseases. I then joined Oxfordshire PCT as a Deputy Director of Public Health, leading on Public Health Strategies and screening and immunisation programmes, before joining Buckinghamshire Public Health team in 2011, where I led on Health Care Public Health and Population Health Management. In 2020, I joined Oxfordshire County Council as a consultant in public health leading on Health Protection, including sexual and reproductive health, cardiovascular disease prevention and the COVID-19 response in Oxfordshire.

I am also an honorary senior clinical lecturer with Oxford University and my academic interests include population health management, reducing inequalities in health outcomes, improving migrants' health and helping older people stay independent in the community.

The challenges and rewards of my current role

Everything about my current job fascinates me. The unpredictability of how my day might begin and end is a constant source of excitement, energy and joy for me. Currently, I lead on Health Protection. A typical week at work includes attending outbreak management meetings, supporting our schools and care homes in preventing infectious disease outbreaks, and ensuring good access to health protection advice and services. I also commission NHS Health Checks and Sexual Health services, and this role varies from undertaking health needs assessments and market testing, to seeking legal and commercial advice, to negotiating service specifications and costs with providers, to finally awarding contracts and managing providers' performance.

Currently, all my work is done in the context of local government. Local government organisations are political bodies, which means that the politicians are in charge. My job as an officer of the council is to provide sound technical advice to them so that their decisions are evidence-based and meet the true needs of our population while recognising their political aspirations – a tricky balance to strike sometimes!

The fact that public health is everyone's business and no single organisation can achieve health alone is a reward as well as a challenge. It is a reward because it guarantees wonderful opportunities to work with people of different backgrounds and with different knowledge and skill-sets and you constantly learn new things. It is a challenge because your success depends on everyone else's cooperation and willingness to play their part and that is where the art of public health come into play. It is those softer skills that you need to use to take everyone with you to form a real partnership and move beyond organisational hierarchy and political boundaries to achieve the greatest good.

Every day brings a new challenge and a new opportunity, and all you need to do your job is your common sense, the core public health skills that you learn during your training and your accumulated experience from doing your job.... oh yes, and a little political nous!

Maintaining a work/life balance

I have always been interested in personal development, be it mental, educational or physical. I do regular exercise to keep fit and read a lot to keep my mind busy and improve my knowledge. The lockdown period during the pandemic provided a wonderful opportunity to read about my new passion, which is British history and politics.

I have a voracious appetite for watching TED Talks[3] and I often start my day by listening to an uplifting speech while getting ready for work.

My contribution to public health

Before the COVID-19 pandemic, as the lead consultant on healthcare public health and population health management, my contribution was mainly around promoting evidence-based medicine and supporting effective and equitable healthcare provision. I ensured that tackling disparities in health and equitable needs-based access to healthcare remained high on the NHS agenda.

As the Chair of Buckinghamshire's statutory multi-agency Child Death Overview Panel, I contributed to preventing avoidable child deaths in Buckinghamshire and supported efforts to safeguard children.

As an educational supervisor, I've contributed to public health training and workforce development and have been privileged to train many public health registrars.

During the pandemic, I led on many aspects of Oxfordshire's response, including coordinating a multi-agency response to COVID-19, developing a local outbreak management plan, setting up COVID-19 testing sites, supporting care homes in managing outbreaks of COVID-19 among vulnerable people and supporting COVID-19 vaccination.

Our response to COVID-19 showcased how the art and science of public health could be brought together to achieve a common goal. A robust surveillance function coupled with strong partnership working were key to bringing the situation under control. For example, the inter- and intra-organisational working particularly between different tiers of local authorities, between local authority and educational settings, between public health and various corporate functions within the council such as Legal, IT, Governance, Customer Services and Finance epitomised real partnership working for health across the system within Oxfordshire.

My ambitions for the future

As far as the future is concerned, I've no fixed plan because not knowing what tomorrow will bring is far more fulfilling and exciting for me. And when it comes to ambition, whenever I'm asked this question, this beautiful quote comes to my mind: 'Be the best version of yourself and let that version shine!' And that is my ambition.

My advice to the next generation

I would like to say three things to the next generation. If you want:

- to change your life for the better;
- to make a difference to other people's lives; and
- to change the world ...

... get involved in public health.

Notes

i According to the World Health Organization, the main determinants of health are the social and economic environment, the physical environment and individual characteristics and behaviours. See Figure 1.1 in Chapter 1 for more.
ii Where different organisations work together formally to plan future projects.
iii See Part 4 for more information about getting started in public health.

References

1. Make Smoking History. *The Cure Project*. Available at: https://thecureproject. co.uk.
2. Marmot, M. *Fair Society, Healthy Lives*, Institute of Health Equity, 2010. Available at: www.instituteofhealthequity.org/resources-reports/fair-society-healthy-lives-the-marmot-review/fair-society-healthy-lives-full-report-pdf.pdf.
3. Free online inspirational/informative/educational talks on a range of topics: www. ted.com/talks.

10 Health policy and system leadership

Jennifer Dixon; David Buck; Durka Dougall; Anne Johnson; Fiona Sim; Jenny Wright

Introduction to this setting

The public health workforce aims to bring about change for the benefit of the population's health and wellbeing. Those working in public health at whatever level, local, regional or national, or beyond, and from whatever organisational base, have to display leadership skills – and often sincere passion – to be able to influence communities, partners and their own and other stakeholder organisations across very complex systems for the benefit of the health of their populations and sometimes for the prevention of serious harm to the health of those populations and communities. Those aiming to influence policymaking are frequently challenging the status quo and provide an objective, evidence-based perspective in addition to political nous and cultural awareness and sensitivity.

They may be employed within the organisation whose policy they aspire to change, or outside, such as in third sector, not-for-profit or non-governmental organisations, or they may be engaged in building the evidence through research in universities.

Challenges and opportunities – vision for health policy and system leadership

Jennifer Dixon, Chief Executive, The Health Foundation

It is hard not to be deeply affected by the searing experience of the COVID-19 pandemic. On the one hand, there was the sight of patients struggling in intensive care, the older person with dementia in a care home unable to see their family, graphs showing the peaks of cases, huge pressure on the NHS and other care services, the analysis showing the differential death rates between the well-off and not-so-well-off, and between ethnic groups. And, of course, by spring 2023, over 227,000 known dead in the UK alone after infection with SARS-CoV-2.

And on the other hand, the marvellous advances of science to produce a vaccine, the rapid testing infrastructure, the jab-rollout, the very hard work of local public health teams working with local organisations to test, trace,

DOI: 10.4324/9781003433699-14

vaccinate and protect, the deeply impressive commitment and application of NHS and care staff, and the leadership of the Chief Medical Officer, Sir Chris Whitty, and many others in public health.

The pandemic was an emergency 'insult' to our health, prompting an emergency response which was complex, dynamic and involving many organisations, public, commercial and charitable. How the response was prepared for and managed will be rightly the subject of reflection in the years to come. The pandemic was rare, and an emergency, but most factors influencing our health are not. They are complex and slow-burn and deserve far greater attention in future. After the pandemic now come other 'insults' to health, not least a cost-of-living crisis and weakened economy, which may have just as profound impacts.

The best estimates are that healthcare has a 10–20% impact on population health. Other factors include so-called 'wider determinants' – support for preschool children, housing, poverty, work, education, air quality, nutrition and so on – which the state largely has responsibility to arrange. We know, for example, there is a gap in health (life expectancy and healthy life expectancy) between those who are well-off and those who aren't, and those living in the north of England and those in the south. In fact, if you did a rough calculation and worked out how many deaths fewer per year there would be if everyone in the country had the same health as those in the top 20%, then the annual figure would be similar to the number of deaths attributable to SARS-CoV-2. We are seared by the impact of the pandemic, but we appear not to be by the similar impact of these wider determinants (on health, and the economy) year in year out. Furthermore, we know from *The Marmot Review: Ten Years On*[1] that since 2011 inequalities in health have grown, that life expectancy is stalling faster in the UK than in most other countries, and that life expectancy has gone into reverse in some parts of the country (less well-off areas in the North East and Midlands, for example). This fraying of the health fabric is also affecting the economy – ill health prevents people from reaching their potential, not least through education and work.

The public health community has long known all this; the question is what to do about it when many look the other way? What should be our vision be and what might leadership in public health achieve? The vision must be to reduce avoidable ill health, have a consistent long-term strategy to improve the 'health capital' of the nation with short-term wins and to work with leaders in other sectors to achieve goals. At national level, this means working to get a proper cross-government strategy to improve population health, including targets, boosting investment and agency in local government, making sure the public health infrastructure and staff at local level are supported and trained, working with business and investors to mobilise action to reduce commercial 'health pollutants' like junk food, poor quality working environments, factory emissions, or online harms, and engaging the public. And as the NHS is Britain's largest 'industry', it means working with national and local NHS bodies to be far more proactive to help reduce risk factors for ill health across populations served. Finally, as the factors influencing health are multiple and interrelated, cast iron scientific evidence on which policies to pursue will be difficult to find. Leaders must be of the highest calibre to be able to use convincing arguments to mobilise action among the many who will use the absence of evidence as a reason for inertia, be fatalistic in the face of a complex challenge, or duck responsibility by focusing blame and agency on individuals who fail to improve their own health.

Championing public health policy and system leadership – two perspectives from The King's Fund

David Buck, Senior Fellow in Public Health and Health Inequalities, and Durka Dougall, Public Health Consultant and Population Health Specialist

David Buck

'An outsider to public health, welcomed in ...'

My journey into, or rather 'around', public health has not been a linear one. I trained as an economist, and after a diversion into defence economics, went to the other end of the spectrum and became a research health economist at the University of York, in the Centre for Health Economics. That's where my interest in, and engagement with, public health started. I applied health economics techniques to public health, in particular to health behaviours such as smoking habits and smoking cessation, and to alcohol use and patterns. Believe it or not, in those days, the tobacco industry was still having some success with economic arguments, and in particular that it supported employment and tax revenue in the UK. One of the most useful pieces of work colleagues and I undertook was to scotch that argument with a piece of analysis looking at what would happen to employment and tax revenue if the then government targets for smoking were met; this combined epidemiological and economic models in creative ways. In short, the money in the economy from spending on smoking would not disappear, but would be spent in different ways and in all likelihood on more labour-intensive goods and services; overall, reducing smoking would be good for employment and the economy.

This sort of experience stimulated my interest in applying economics and other techniques to real-world policy problems. From there, by way of a short period teaching health economics to dental students at Guy's Hospital in the Department of Dental Public Health, I was lucky enough to apply for and get a job in the Department of Health as an economic adviser. That role was broad and varied, including making the case for more preventive diabetes care. It led to other more strategic and policy roles, including on childhood obesity, stints seconded into other parts of government including the prime minister's forward strategy unit and, latterly, in helping to deliver government commitments on health inequalities reduction.

Since the beginning of 2011, upon leaving government, I have worked for The King's Fund. We are a charity and 'think-tank' at the intersection of policy, research and practice with a goal of improving health and care for all. This has given me the opportunity to take the learning, experience and networks and apply them in new ways and develop them further. Prime among that has been a stronger focus on working with local health and care systems and others, including the role of local government public health teams. It's also given me the space to develop thinking with others, including Durka, on approaches to improving population health and to help support local areas make sense of that and put it into practice; to develop my understanding of the role of the voluntary and community sector in health; and to be a critical friend and constructive thorn-in-the-side of colleagues in government. Most recently, I have had the privilege of documenting and sharing for a wider audience some of the activities and challenges of being a Director of Public Health in the time of COVID-19.

So, to draw together some thoughts on my journey 'into' public health ... The key thing for me is that there are many ways in and routes to working for the public's health, whether that's through formal training programmes, research, direct delivery of care and preventive services, or policy or other ways. The key thing is to find your own way: for some, that will be based on a plan of attack known in advance; for others, including me, it will be a meandering journey collecting experiences, learning and benefiting from the generosity of many others along the way, and recognising and taking chances when they arrive. But if you do join the journey, you will be assured of a welcome and a family of people all contributing to, and motivated by, the same core goal: to help improve the health of the population. That's not a bad journey to start out on.

Durka Dougall

'Building Capability across UK for Improving Health and Tackling Health Inequalities'

Public health practice – purpose

There may be a temptation to see public health simply as a career option, or maybe a set of three functions: health protection, health promotion, health-care public health. The reality is that it is so much more. The commonly used definition of public health by Acheson gives a sense of this breadth, describing public health as: 'the art and science of preventing disease, prolonging life and promoting health through the organized efforts of society'.[2] If we see public health in this broader sense, it is a purpose; where many people – those who would say they work in public health, and many who wouldn't – all play an important part. For me, the deep understanding of this is something that has developed over a 25-year career across a variety of roles. It is this that lies at the heart of my current work as an accredited public health specialist and medical practitioner working to improve population health across the UK. There is an interesting debate about the overlap between population health and public health; depending on your viewpoint, this will vary. But one thing is clear: public health is essential for population health efforts. There are countless examples of good practice already across various sectors (for example, community, charity, NHS, education, council, social care, transport, policing, integrated care systems, primary care networks, industry and more). There also exists potential to improve people's health and tackle health inequalities even more by joining up efforts across these different organisations and sectors; in particular by supporting people across a variety of roles and sectors, whether individuals (from boards to frontline staff), teams (regardless of size), organisations (from many sectors) and systems (multi-agency groupings), to help them see their contribution for improving population health and to take steps to realise this in practice jointly with others. This became the focus of my work.

Why this matters

Working as a medical doctor, I saw first-hand the need for more proactive, prevention-focused and whole-systems ways of working. As a surgeon, I found myself caring for patients who did not always need to be in hospital. It was not evident when caring for their symptoms and thinking about their immediate medical needs. But when I took time to hear their stories, I spotted missed opportunities for preventive care, early input, timely support in the community, removing unnecessary gaps and indeed better joins in the care for patients after surgery. There were times when we could not discharge people from hospital due to system fragments; barriers accessing care packages or safe transfer back to the community. I saw that often the most vulnerable people suffered the most from this – something that is widely recognised in the literature around health inequalities. I wanted to do something about this, and as I looked more into it, I started to realise that other staff felt similarly. I saw that people (staff and communities) had tremendous potential to help bring about improvements when given the right support – far more than I as an individual could ever have alone when trying to make improvements to health and care. I realised that the greatest opportunity was in enabling others to unlock their potentials for improving health and care. That is when I came across the concepts of systems leadership, quality improvement, population health and public health – over time, I undertook training in all of these.

My system improvement interest took me to a career as a healthcare commissioner in a primary care trust and I marvelled at the sheer amount that I found possible even with limited funds by just applying some basic principles. Whether in the design of an aortic aneurysm screening programme across a region, or rolling out a national HPV vaccination (human papilloma virus vaccine against cervical cancer and other cancers), understanding the needs of the most vulnerable communities in a highly deprived area, tackling primary care variation across a whole borough or supporting educational reform across a sector, it was clear that, with positive support, practical guidance, a collaborative approach and sustained efforts, much was possible. In my spare time, I began work as a non-executive member of the board of a mental health charity and through this learned the real power of whole-systems approaches. I saw that many partners such as charities offer a tremendous amount to the improvement of health and it was remarkable to see what is possible through wide-reaching effective partnership.

So, I trained as a public health specialist, working initially in a local authority and then in the NHS. I now work as a Senior Consultant and Programme Director at The King's Fund. I'm also a clinical academic affiliated to two universities (University College London and University of East London) and a volunteer supporting school children from deprived communities to access medical careers. My work, often in collaboration with colleagues like Dave and others, focuses on helping people to consider their role also in public health and population health, and to help them to maximise their contribution to improving the health and care of others. Despite doing this for over five years and having trained over 800 people in population health during this time, I never cease to be amazed by the sheer potential that can be unlocked when individuals, teams, organisations and systems are supported well to do this. I have worked with boards of hospitals and integrated care trusts, helped regions to set up academies for Population Health and Equity, led on the training of whole workforce groupings across sectors, and helped people at individual levels to take their own next steps wherever they are to improving health and tackling health inequalities. I feel very proud of what has been achieved and feel so lucky to have worked with so many wonderful people from across health and care along the way. It feels like a real step change is beginning in this area and there is just huge potential from it having been taken even thus far. But I can also see how much more is needed to achieve the aspiration to provide the best possible health and care for everyone; and the challenges that yet lay ahead to do this well. Hence the importance for me in writing this for you. Because as you think about your career, I hope you too will think about your role in helping to deliver this.

My top three tips

My best advice to you is first and foremost to start with purpose. Why are you doing what you are doing? What are you hoping to achieve? For whom? Second – be true to yourself. A supervisor told me a long while ago: 'Be the best you that you can be. You don't need to be like anyone else. Focus on being the best version of yourself that you can possibly be.' Third – enjoy the journey. If you do decide to pursue a career in public health, you will find public health to be a most enjoyable, flexible, exciting and rewarding career and one that I would certainly recommend. And if you decide to pursue something different, regardless of what you choose, hopefully you will now see that whoever you are, in whichever role, you can also play an important role in helping to ensure the best possible health and care for everyone.

Career story

Anne Johnson, Professor of Epidemiology and Director of Centre of Infectious Disease Epidemiology, University College London and President of the Academy of Medical Sciences

How I first became interested in public health

This takes me back to my days as an undergraduate in medicine at Cambridge University. I applied to go there rather than to a classical medical school because of the opportunity to study a different subject in my third undergraduate year – in my case, social and political sciences. Looking at the social determinants of health made me realise that health was not driven just by medical interventions. This was consolidated by a gap year in Venezuela after graduation, when I was not sure that I still wanted to do medicine. In South America I saw – writ large – immense disparities in health between the oil rich and those living in 'barrios' (informal settlements), as well as the impact of introduction of infectious diseases on isolated, indigenous populations. This gave me the opportunity to reflect on the challenge and ethics of improving health globally. It has influenced me throughout my career.

Returning to the UK in 1975, I embarked on my clinical medical course, subsequently training as a GP in Newcastle. General practice is a good way to learn about public health: I saw at first hand people's lives and jobs and their home circumstances in Northumbrian mining towns. My training included a Community Medicine placement with the Riverside child health project working with deprived communities and I did my first research project on undetected squints in children. I also had a chance to do an epidemiology course – a revelation at the time.

Getting trained in public health and starting an academic career

I had discovered public health as a career and gained a place on the Community Medicine training scheme in North East London in 1983. I completed my Master's at the London School of Hygiene and Tropical Medicine in 1984. My summer project involved working in the refugee camps of Thailand and Malaysia on sexual violence towards migrating Vietnamese 'boat people', cementing my interest in women's health.

I wanted an academic career, but it was hard to persuade service public health colleagues of its merits. An introduction to Mike Adler (then Professor of Genitourinary Medicine) changed my career. He was looking for a lecturer trained in public health to research sexually transmitted infections (STIs) and

HIV. This led to a two-year lectureship with Mike and June Crown (later President of the Faculty of Public Health). I started work at the Middlesex Hospital Medical School in 1985, which later became part of University College London (UCL). I have been there ever since.

Some colleagues at the time said working on AIDS (which had been first described in 1981) would ruin my career. We forget now, but there was so much stigma against those infected with HIV at that time, and those presenting with an AIDS diagnosis had an average life-expectancy of six months. The gay community led the early AIDS prevention campaigns, including promoting 'safe sex' (a new term then) and the use of condoms. I saw both the severe impact of the epidemic and the mobilisation of the gay community in response in 1986 on a King's Fund Fellowship trip to San Francisco and New York.

Climbing the academic, and starting on the policy, ladder

Once back in the UK, I was funded, with Mike Adler and David Miller at St Mary's Hospital, to establish the MRC UK Coordinating Centre for HIV/AIDS epidemiological research. Among my first work was an investigation into whether and how HIV could be transmitted between heterosexual couples. This was the start of a career studying STI and HIV epidemiology. The HIV epidemic was being driven by patterns of sexual behaviour and injecting drug use, but virtually nothing was known about this at population level. This really hampered projections and models of likely HIV spread, as well as the services needed for prevention and care. In 1990, I led, with a team of colleagues, the first of the large-scale random sample surveys on sexual behaviour – the National Survey of Sexual Attitudes and Lifestyle (NATSAL). In the 1980s, the concept of sexual health did not exist. There were questions we did not know the answers to – what fraction of the population had same-sex partners, how many partners did people have, what was the pattern of sexual practices and what proportion of people injected recreational drugs? To answer these questions, we needed to look at the pattern of behaviour across the whole population. People thought it was a bit crazy attempting to do this. But with careful preparatory work on how to ask questions, how to protect people's privacy, and emphasising the public health importance of the topic, we found that people took it seriously, and we achieved a 65% response rate from a random sample survey of nearly 19,000 people. This first survey hit the headlines even before it got into the field and was famously banned from public funding by the then Prime Minister, Margaret Thatcher, but, thankfully, was subsequently funded by the Wellcome Trust, with the first results published in *Nature* magazine in 1992. Two further surveys followed in 2000 and 2010, and a fourth is now in progress. Over the years, the surveys have informed policy on HIV services, sex education, contraception, chlamydia and HPV vaccination among many other topics. NATSAL has become a big resource and is probably the largest and most detailed series of sample surveys on sexual lifestyles in the world.

In 1998, I took a sabbatical in Australia with my family, returning to UCL to set up the Centre for Disease Epidemiology, which Andrew Hayward (now Director of the UCL Institute of Epidemiology and Health Care) subsequently joined. Alongside the sexual health work, in 2007 we established the Medical Research Council (MRC) funded 'Flu Watch' to study the epidemiology of influenza in a large representative community sample. Then, in 2009, a new flu strain emerged, which could possibly have become a serious pandemic. We were able to demonstrate through our cohort survey that the new pandemic virus was, in fact, less virulent than had been initially feared and that the majority of flu infections caused mild or no symptoms, and we were able to understand some of the biological factors that protect people from severe disease.

By that time, my management responsibilities were increasing and, in 2002, I became Head of Department and later Head of Division, and became interested in science policy. I served on Medical Research Council (MRC) panels and chaired the public health group, serving on the Strategy Board. Then the Wellcome Trust advertised for governors for its Board. It was a long shot, but I was appointed in 2011 and served for eight years – a fascinating experience and an opportunity to contribute to science strategy and funding in an increasingly international organisation.

Broadening the scope

My work on HIV got me interested in global health issues and, in 2007, with Anthony Costello, we established the UCL Institute for Global Health as a cross-university initiative. One of our first pieces of work was the first ever Lancet Commission on Health and Climate Change, a precursor to the Lancet Countdown on Health and Climate Change. This later gave me the opportunity to serve as a member of the Adaptation Sub-Committee of the UK Climate Change Committee, providing a new opportunity to contribute cross-disciplinary scientific advice to government.

My most recent leadership roles

When I left the Wellcome Trust in 2019, I was appointed Vice President of the Academy of Medical Sciences (AMS), one of four independent UK academies (the others being the British Academy, the Royal Society and the Royal Academy of Engineering). I had enjoyed working previously with AMS, chairing the Academy's Working Group for the 2016 report on 'Improving the Health of the Public by 2040'. The report emphasised the critical need for transdisciplinary research to improve public health and particularly the 'upstream' drivers. This needed a much wider base of research – for example, from economists, lawyers, behavioural scientists and those studying the built and natural environment. AMS was able to bring together a multidisciplinary group of scientists from different backgrounds, most of them AMS Fellows, to develop the report.

The report influenced the establishment of the UK Committee for Strategic Coordination of Health of the Public Research (SCHOPR), which I chair, and which is a sub-board of the Office for Strategic Coordination of Health Research (OSCHR). It is a committee of funders which considers how to optimise research investment and has, for example, advised the four UK Chief Medical Officers on priorities. A key area has been to develop research on prevention, not only into the health service, but in local government. Public health colleagues rightly challenge academics to ask more relevant questions for public health practice, to provide evidence of effective interventions and not just describe problems. COVID-19 has really highlighted increasing health inequalities, while all of us face the global existential challenges of climate change, environmental damage and the consequences of conflict. A big challenge for the future is to ensure, therefore, that those in academia work more closely with practitioners on the ground, so that they ask and answer the right questions and produce relevant research evidence to benefit population health. But, for this to happen, we need more secure careers for public health researchers and more appropriate investment in transdisciplinary research. The National Institute of Health and Care Research (NIHR) and others are now investing in some exciting new career schemes alongside the multi-funder Prevention Research Programme coordinated by the MRC. But there is much more to be done and I hope that the new public health organisations in England, including the UK Health Security Agency (UKHSA) and the Office for Health Improvement and Disparities (OHID), will work to develop stronger research capability in partnership with academic colleagues.

The COVID-19 pandemic provided a new impetus for my career. I was drawn into the AMS response on COVID-19, ranging from advice to UK Research and Innovation (UKRI) and others on research funding, serving on a sub-group of the Scientific Advisory Group for Emergencies (SAGE) and working on several reports, including the AMS report 'Preparing for a challenging winter', commissioned by Sir Patrick Vallance, the government's Chief Scientific Advisor. And I had to hone my media skills as broadcast and print media became increasingly thirsty for epidemiologists to comment.

Why I am an epidemiologist

I didn't really know about public health until I had lessons in epidemiology at Newcastle. I found it provided a different perspective on how diseases are distributed in the population and what determines them, and then how to use that evidence to guide action. How you could, for example, work out the link between smoking and cancer, but also the wide range of work needed to disseminate that evidence and use it to drive prevention policy. I wanted to understand the causes and prevention of diseases. My time at the London School of Hygiene and Tropical Medicine gave me an understanding of epidemiology – and then HIV came along. In researching infectious diseases, we also had to put together social, economic behavioural, environmental and public perspectives.

Reflecting on my career

Throughout my career in academia and public health, I have always had an eye on the big picture. This provided the opportunity to work on policy and the evidence base for policy, trying to enable effective public health interventions whatever the politics of the day.

My proudest achievement

I take an immense pleasure in seeing the next generation thrive and take on the new challenges with new approaches. For example, I am no longer an investigator for NATSAL and the team who have taken on the latest survey have brought new ideas and novel scientific approaches. It is great to see something I started continuing and which has helped people in their careers just as I was encouraged by others early in my career. When they stop asking for my advice, it will be time to step aside!

I am also proud of being involved in founding a specific niche area, which now people respect as an important area of medicine and health, and which has broadened out immensely from our initial concerns of HIV to the wider field of sexual health.

Advice to the next generation

I did not plan my career, but I did look for, and take, opportunities for whatever fired my imagination. It has been a combination of serendipity and hard work on the way. Follow your heart, but use your head to get there.

References

1. Professor Sir Michael Marmot. *Health Equity in England: The Marmot Review 10 Years On*, The Health Foundation, February 2020. Available at: www.health. org.uk/publications/reports/the-marmot-review-10-years-on.
2. Acheson, D. *Public Health in England: The Report of the Committee of Inquiry into the Future Development of the Public Health Function*, Cm 209, London, HMSO, 1988.

11 UK voluntary and community sector

Shirley Cramer; Andrew Evans;
Joanne Bosanquet; Fiona Sim;
Jenny Wright

Introduction to this setting

Voluntary and community sector (VCS) organisations, including charities, have been working to improve the health of the population for many centuries both in the UK and overseas. Increasingly, they are being used to deliver direct core care as well as supplement the work of statutory agencies such as, in the UK, the NHS and local government. They often play a major role in advocacy for the cause they represent, sometimes working in partnership with other like-minded organisations to lobby politicians in support of their shared priorities. Public health roles will vary, but some of the very large charities will look to public health professionals to undertake leadership roles, but also data analysis, research including explaining the evidence-base, policy and document preparation and communication to key organisations and policy makers as well as the general public.

Challenges and opportunities – vision for the voluntary and community sector's contribution to public health

Shirley Cramer, former Chief Executive, the Royal Society for Public Health

As we emerge from the COVID-19 pandemic, it is clear that our public health indicators have gone in the wrong direction. This is probably not surprising given the length and severity of the pandemic and the poor condition of the nation's health as we entered the COVID-19 era in 2020. More than ten years of austerity had left most local authorities and the NHS barely able to cope with the urgent in health and care, let alone the necessary preventive programmes and structural changes to ensure a healthy and equal nation.

In 2022, our health inequalities are writ large. We have an ageing population, along with one of the oldest housing stocks in Europe, a fragile welfare state, vast inequalities in jobs and education, unequal access to food and increasing obesity, inadequate transport and insufficient high quality early years' services. We have a 19 years' difference in healthy life expectancy between the poorest and the wealthiest in the UK, despite having a universal

DOI: 10.4324/9781003433699-15

healthcare system which, in theory, should support us all equally. But we know it's not just about healthcare, don't we? Mortality rates for COVID-19 were more than twice as high from the 10% most deprived local areas and significantly worse for those from the Black and minority ethnic (BME) communities, compared with the country as a whole.

So what is the future of public health? Although inequalities are significantly worse, they are also more visible and, most importantly, the population is concerned about them. Even before the Conservatives' 'Partygate' scandal had fuelled a 'them and us' narrative, public polling by the Health Foundation showed that 55% were concerned that COVID-19 had worsened health inequalities and eight in ten people agreed that government must address unequal outcomes.

So does an increased awareness of the disparities in our society and the government's recent 'levelling up' plan for England (2022) provide an opportunity? The social determinants of health should be addressed through the levelling up plan, highlighting as it does the strategy proposed by Sir Michael Marmot.[1] But, as he has pointed out, the level of ambition requires a large investment in funding, which is so far missing.

Another small sign for optimism is the recognition that inequality is embedded in our current structures and environment. This is an important change. One of the reasons that we have made little progress in improving the public's health is the ideology of individual responsibility. It is 'your fault' if you smoke, you are obese, have a marginal job, are hungry or live in inadequate housing. Researchers at the University of Cambridge showed that from 1993 to 2015 we had 689 separate obesity policies and yet, over this time, obesity rose among adults from 15% to 27%. For three decades, we have had similar and failing policies, when we know that these issues are determined to a large extent by environmental factors, and our failure to tackle structural issues such as ultra-processed food.

There is a real role for the third sector in holding the government's feet to the fire on the levelling up plan and campaigning for proper funding. We should aim to follow the example of New Zealand and include health and wellbeing across all departments and measure progress regularly. In this way, public health is a national priority. This approach, which has been demonstrated in Wales by the Future Generations Act of 2015, supports long-term outcomes and a prevention strategy.

We already know that the voluntary sector was critical during the pandemic, organising locally, coordinating volunteers and developing services where the need was greatest – whether this was food banks or supporting the vaccine rollout. The use of the wider workforce across the voluntary sector to support health improvement is already widespread, ensuring the widest possible responsibility for health and wellbeing, and this will need to be expanded in the next few years.

Increased local autonomy on a range of issues with funding to support it would enable local authorities and the voluntary sector to work with local communities to drive forward policies and programmes that they all agree with.

Overview of the voluntary and community sector as a public health setting

Andrew Evans, Chief Executive Officer of the charity METRO

An overview of the setting

The VCS is vibrant, agile, buoyant and able to respond to a crisis and meet the community's needs at its doorstep. While the statutory sector services are often centrally located, the number and diversity of VCSs we have in our cities and towns means we deliver public health work directly into a community. There are fewer barriers for individuals to accessing services in the community, such as travel, associated costs and time. As a sector, we work extremely hard to build the respect and trust of our communities, which is paramount in our work and informs the approaches we take. By respecting the individual, culture and community, we collaborate with leaders and key stakeholders to find mutual goals and objectives. For example, at METRO we have worked with local faith leaders and Imams to facilitate conversations with congregations and communities that encourage HIV testing to take place.

An added strength of the sector is that staff and volunteers often have an affiliation with the aims and objectives of the charity, meaning they are regularly peers, and consequently have a deeper understanding of the core issues. Peer work is immensely powerful in voluntary and community settings and is often a further strength of our work. We regularly find that seeing people like yourself, achieving goals you may aspire to, can be uplifting and encouraging for individuals and create a desire for attainment that is possible and realistic.

The sector is also valuable in supporting vulnerable clients who may have built up distrust or fear of the statutory or NHS services. For example, at METRO, our first community HIV testing clinic, Pitstops Clinic for men who have sex with men, regularly attracted people too nervous and anxious to attend a hospital Genitourinary Medicine (GUM) clinic. We also use our volunteers and community assets to actively seek out and engage those in need of support, and use these connections to encourage positive health behaviours.

The sector

VCS organisations come in all shapes and sizes, from small volunteer-led groups with little to no funding to multinational multimillion-pound organisations. METRO Charity started in 1984 as a small charity called the Greenwich Lesbian and Gay Centre, campaigning for lesbian and gay rights in the community, and for many years solely worked with LGBTQ+[i] people. However, in 2008, we changed our constitution to say that, as a charity, we will support any person experiencing issues related to sexuality, equality, diversity and identity. We operate across five domains: Sexual and Reproductive Health, Community, Mental Health and Wellbeing, Youth and HIV. We have a turnover of approximately £5 million, employ 90 staff and work with 70 volunteers to provide services and campaigns across London and the South East of England. The sector is dependent on outside funding from various sources, including trusts and foundations, local authority, individual giving and corporate sponsors. At METRO, we rely on various funding sources and regularly work in partnership with other charities and NHS Trusts to bid for contracts and grants to deliver services. One of these services is our METRO GAVS programme,[2] where we support Greenwich's local voluntary and not-for-profit sectors in governance, finance and fundraising.

VCS organisations are often creative and flexible when deciding where to work, often using several settings and, in many cases, relying on clients to tell us where they feel most comfortable. For example, outreach services to engage young people will often happen after school and early evening at venues such as skate parks and/or near fast-food outlets. Libraries are also extensively used as they are community settings, can reduce any stigma associated with getting support and are regularly accessible. Many services are also delivered in the home, or close to home, where the person feels the most comfortable. In this way, our role is to reduce barriers the individual may have and create the optimal atmosphere to facilitate a positive intervention and experience of care.

Throughout all this, it is important to remember that VCS organisations are workplaces. While everyone may feel passionate about the aims and goals of the organisation, we still have all the same workplace and interpersonal challenges as any other workplace in the public or private sector. As a sector, we must constantly combat inequities within the system, including racism, disablism, ageism, misogyny, homophobia, biphobia, and transphobia, and ensure sufficient diversity in our workforce.

The likely impact of imminent NHS reforms in England

In the first instance, I believe the 2022 changes will favour larger charities that can support Integrated Care Systems (ICS) leadership with paid time, as part of their business model of understanding the changes in the landscape. Smaller charities, made up of a majority volunteer staff base, will find it difficult to spend the time needed to understand the changes or join in system-level meetings. Consequently, there will be those who benefit more than others and it will be up to the ICS to engage with the VCS in a meaningful and comprehensive way. The reforms' impact will depend on how well they understand the makeup of the new ICS and Integrated Care Boards (ICBs), how integrated they are into the decision-making, and whether they can respond to the opportunities quickly and efficiently when they become available.

Local government and the NHS have seen that the VCS is integral to public health, but funding to support organisations by local government has reduced. There is, for example, a need for Black and minority ethnic-led VSC organisations to be properly resourced so they can drive and lead the ideas and implement effective approaches for the communities they reflect.

VCS organisations' contribution to public health

Regardless of the charity, public health has always been what the VCS does, even when the aims and objectives may be focused on support for animals or nature, the act of volunteering and working in the community has positive mental health benefits being recognised by the NHS. The recent COVID-19 pandemic is a good example of how the sector contributes to public health and the government's realisation of how dependent the system is on our contribution. Many more vulnerable people and communities would have suffered if it were not for the many thousands of volunteer hours that supported the response. While in early April 2022, the Chancellor provided £750 million to support the sector through the pandemic, we equally helped the local and national infrastructure across the country to support those in need. Locally in the Royal Borough of Greenwich, organisations like Charlton Athletic Community Trust and Volunteer Centre Greenwich (VCG) organised food parcels to be delivered to vulnerable people, while METRO worked with clients to provide hardship grants and advocacy around benefits and support. As in many areas across the country, the local volunteer centre, VCG, was also integral in providing volunteers to deliver the vaccination rollout across the borough.

The VCS also had an essential role in reflecting to local authorities and public health professionals the impact COVID-19 was having on specific communities – for example, Black and minority ethnic communities, people living with HIV, LGBTQ+ young people living in toxic households where their sexuality or gender identity was not respected, disabled people, and those with mental health support needs. At the start of the pandemic, METRO's research group collated data from across the charity, highlighting the disproportionate impact COVID-19 had on people with intersecting protected characteristics and submitted evidence to the Women and Equalities Parliamentary Select Committee Inquiry in late April 2020. Twelve months on, METRO again evaluated the impact COVID was having on our clients and shared these findings as a report, which can be found on our website.[3]

Current methodologies employ a population health approach which, according to The King's Fund, is an approach that aims to improve physical and mental health outcomes, promote wellbeing and reduce health inequalities across an entire population. This involves acknowledging that the wider determinants of health (for example, income, education, housing, employment, etc.) are significant factors in shaping the health of a community. Consequently, we, as health professionals, must listen to and work with the community to create changes to improve health that will be achievable and sustainable. Co-production is vital in ensuring services are built so they directly respond to the community's needs. The VCS can often act as advocates

and facilitate communication between the local community and local authority and/or NHS to help create programmes from the ground up. As a sector,
we can also be a critical friend to councils and the NHS and support in
evaluation and monitoring through the promotion of functions such as client
advisory panels and service user groups.

An example of community collaboration with the NHS from METRO's history dates from the early 2000s, when HIV and STI testing among men who
have sex with men (MSM) was still medicalised, with recommendations from
organisations such as NICE that all MSM should only be seen in GUM clinics. However, we knew there were various reasons, including fear and stigma,
which prevented many MSM from attending GUM clinics for HIV testing.
As a result, in 2001, METRO collaborated with the local GUM clinic at the
Queen Elizabeth Hospital to open one of the first HIV testing clinics outside of
a GUM setting in the form of a satellite clinic. This approach attracted many
first-time HIV testers because of the non-clinical and community environment
provided by the charity, and was supported by volunteer clinic hosts.

A myriad of public health roles and career opportunities

There are many public health roles in the VCS with various positions on
offer – for example, management, front-line work, support work, strategy,
research or IT. Each charity has a unique mission statement and values,
which will give candidates a good sense of its core direction and can therefore
establish if they match their own passion and interests. Research charities
that pique your interest, as there will always be one that matches your skills,
experience and passion, and look for ways to get involved.

You can often start in smaller ways as a part-time volunteer, which allows you to get accustomed to the sector and the people within it. You might
browse job websites like The Third Sector, *The Guardian* or Charity Jobs,
and you can often do this by sector, level and location (from local to international), for voluntary or paid work. If you are developing your skills in a
particular area, you might seek courses where placements in the sector are
part of the course. These can give you a feel for the work environment in a
way that can enhance your learning experience.

There are many skills that VCS organisations are looking for, especially
around data, data analytics, IT and communications, but be aware they are
often not remunerated at private sector levels. However, there are benefits
other than pay that the VCS organisations often provide as part of their support and investment in their staff and the wider workforce, so look out for
these and make your own assessment.

Qualities and skills needed

You will need a certain amount of resilience to work in the sector as there
is a lot of internal and external change that can impact the charity, and

consequently employment. Most VCS organisations have a small funding base which, even with careful management, can be uncertain and change as priorities change with funders, local authorities or individual givers. Staff contracts are often aligned with contracts that are successfully tendered for, which means there can be a fair amount of movement when contracts change hands and staff potentially move via TUPE (Transfer of Undertakings – Protection of Employment). Hence, having a versatile approach to applying your skills and abilities is really beneficial as you may be offered, or need to apply for, new and varied roles if and when contracts change.

Even beyond the contractual changes, the innovative approaches we need to take to engage with communities to improve our reach and impact means developing your skills and applying them to different situations will significantly enhance what you can achieve. Being open to change, accepting new ways of communicating (such as using non-binary pronouns they/them) and embracing technology (such as using Twitter/Instagram) will help streamline and make you more efficient and effective in what you do. However, many of our most vulnerable clients won't be online or on Twitter, or even using Facebook, so ensuring you continue reaching and working with these individuals remains a priority.

The challenges and rewards of my role

After being with the charity for 20 years in many various positions, I have only recently been appointed CEO and, therefore, I am still quite new to the role. After being at the charity as long as I have, I have just started an induction schedule that feels really refreshing and will enable me to look at the charity through a different lens. In the short time that I've officially been CEO, I've definitely felt a change in the depth of the responsibility and the potential impact decisions I make can have on a day-to-day basis. This can be particularly challenging as competing priorities are presented, all completely valid in merit, but decisions may, in turn, favour one area over another. The cost-of-living crisis is a challenge for charities, staff are finding it tough and contracts made on costings based on prices 12 to 24 (and longer) months ago are redundant in the current climate.

Despite the challenges, it's an exciting time to lead a charity such as METRO, with the goals and aspirations that can truly impact people's lives. We have a vibrant and engaged staff team that are very dedicated to our thousands of clients, and as a leadership team, we work together to better invest and shape the charity's leadership.

An example of my charity's contribution to public health

There are many examples of METRO's contribution to public health from our five domains – from supporting LGBTQ+ young people, to counselling, to supporting those living with or affected by HIV. One contribution METRO has championed particularly is the provision of free condoms and Chlamydia screening for young people across South London and the South East.

As a charity, we were one of the first to provide young people 16 years and over with access to condoms via an online ordering and postal service.

The implementation of the National Chlamydia Screening Programme (NCSP) in 2008 meant millions of Chlamydia screening tests were sent to young people via GP registration lists, but there was a huge reluctance by the statutory sector to send condoms separately or with the kits. There was a perception that providing condoms encourages sex, particularly for underage people. Those responsible appeared more concerned about receiving criticism from parents than providing sexual health support. This, coupled with guidelines that placed several other barriers for young people to accessing condoms, made me terribly frustrated. Therefore, we created 'Get it', an online condom website. In Kent and Medway, we have seen great improvements in accessing condoms: since 2014, in Kent, there have been 29,000 registrations and 67,000 orders and in Medway 10,000 registrations. The model is now being introduced into some South London boroughs.

My own career journey

My journey illustrates you do not need to be formally trained in public health or have public health in your job title to have a role in improving health outcomes in the community. In fact, the National Council for Voluntary Organisations (NCVO) estimate there are three million volunteers working in health in the UK, which I would say are all supporting public health.

I moved to the UK from Australia in 1998 for a gap year during my teaching degree and ended up staying. Initially, I spent three years in Bristol before moving to London in 2001. In Australia, I'd volunteered at the AIDS Council of New South Wales (ACON) and was looking for something similar to do in London to meet friends who had similar interests, engage in the LGBTQ+ community and support change. I found an advert in a local paper for volunteers at The Metro Centre and applied to be a gay men's outreach volunteer on health promotion work. My early experiences were of many late nights giving out condoms in bars across South East London and demystifying what happened at sexual health clinics to encourage attendance.

Between 2005 and 2010, while working part-time at METRO as a gay men's outreach worker, I was also director of my own company, which delivered face-to-face fundraising for charities at events and venues they managed. When I moved to full-time work with METRO, I closed the company and eventually became Metro's Director of Health and Community Services, a post I held for several years.

I have completed several training programmes on the way, with my Master's completed relatively late in my career in 2016, but giving me additional perspective and skills I would never have acquired had I been younger.

Advice to anyone considering doing public health in this sector

Public health is an exciting and ever-moving landscape. People change and develop, and technology improves, so we have endless opportunities to create and innovate across several competencies.

My advice? Find the cause/organisation that you are passionate about and reach out.

Career story

Joanne Bosanquet, Chief Executive Officer, Foundation of Nursing Studies

Public health is ingrained in my DNA

I am often asked when I knew I wanted to be a nurse. When I was young, I was genuinely interested in people and communities. I grew up in a colliery village in South Yorkshire in a blend of a middle- and working-class family. I remember my father being on strike from the pits in 1986 and he lost nearly everything, but stayed on strike. This instilled in me that one should do the right thing for the right reasons. I was really into advocacy and wanted society to be better and fairer. A sense of justice was deeply ingrained from a young age. My mother was a teacher who also did night school and summer school. She had an enormous work ethic – she worked all the time. It taught me to be self-sufficient from a young age too. My life was a bit chaotic. I was an angry teenager! I didn't like school and did not find the O-levels and CSEs[ii] on offer at all exciting, so became disenfranchised, leaving school at 16 with nothing. Then, because my mother worked at the local college, a colleague of hers suggested I could join the 16–18 access course on health and social care. It was a pre-nursing course in Doncaster and I studied O-levels that weren't available at school, such as sociology, psychology and human development. I loved it and it opened up my world!

Qualifying and working as a nurse

It was when I saw the Hillsborough[iii] tragedy on television I knew I had to work in the sector. There was no plan B (apart from a hankering to be an actress in musical theatre, which is still there!).

When I was 18, I moved onto nurse training in Sheffield. The training was very varied, lots of different hospitals – old tuberculosis (TB) hospitals and Nightingale wards.[iv] Matrons and ward sisters were in charge. On the medical wards there were men with chest, heart and vascular conditions whose life expectancy was poor. It was an industrial city. I saw it again and again. I started to ask questions: how had they ended up in hospital, why did they need amputations? It was the late 1980s, before there was an emphasis on long-term conditions, and there was no attention paid to lifestyles. They all smoked – as did the nurses! We used to take patients out for a cigarette. We didn't think about it!

During my training, I learned a lot about people and loved the technical stuff, but felt hemmed in on the wards. I also asked too many questions and there was nobody to talk to me about it. I got frustrated. I was young, 21, so when I qualified I tried theatres and A&E, then anaesthetics. I found a course in London and became an anaesthetic nurse at St Mary's Hospital, where I saw lots of stabbings and trauma. I did this for two years, but again felt hemmed in. Although I had my nursing registration, I had no degree. I didn't even have A-levels, so at the age of 26 I decided I would give it a go. I worked for a nursing agency for three years while studying full time for a degree in health studies at North London University, now London Metropolitan University. I even got funded as a mature student. It allowed me to focus on health, wellness and society and filled in some knowledge gaps. In fact, it blew my head off! I loved it – looking at policy, politics and communities. Some lecturers were activists and many were left-wing. I am still in contact with some of them now.

Life as a health visitor

I met a student on the degree programme who was studying for a post-regis-tration qualification in health visiting. I knew nothing about health visiting – I had been told it was all twinsets and pearls! She suggested I came to work with her one day. My mind was open – all those mothers and babies and the sophisticated verbal communication that was going on with them. So I went to King's College straight after my degree in 1999 to study for a post-graduate diploma in health visiting. I found the academic side quite challenging – too traditional for someone who had a left-wing view of the world. I always had my arm up for questions that were often left unanswered. Yet, practising as a student health visitor in the Hasidic Jewish community in north London taught me how to approach and embrace different cultures. One thing the King's course had taught me was how to undertake a community needs as-sessment, so I did one on my patch, spent a lot of time in the library looking at Office for National Statistics (ONS) and census data, then took them to the local Director of Public Health – student health visitors or even nurses did not go and see their local Directors of Public Health! My first question was why did he not have a nurse on his team? I ended up doing a bit of work with the public health department. Through this, I met Professor Ros Bryar of City University, who asked me to get involved with some work on the future of nursing in Hackney. I qualified and spent the next 18 months or so in a very deprived part of Hackney. My caseload was extremely varied and I could write a book just on my experiences during this time!

In 2002, I got a job in Doncaster as a specialist health visitor working with refugees and asylum seekers – they were literally being bused up north from the south! It was a Primary Medical Services (PMS) pilot and a colleague, Ka-ren, and myself ran it from a tiny office. We employed a salaried doctor. One day, a number of coaches arrived at the same time with people from all over the world. It was going to take weeks to go through their lived experiences. I was out of my depth – where to start? My Mum suggested I talk to the chaplain at her college, which I did, and I realised what they needed was kinship, or a religious community, some place to identify with, which we sorted for them. It was an important public health lesson – find out what people need, don't tell them. I also linked up with the local Director of Public Health and we set up a proper policy for the TB and contact tracing service. In this job, I learned about negotiation, nudging, bargaining – when you are communicating over something which is not the other person's priority. We worked with interpreters, but it was incredibly complex. My colleague and I met with local charities to get the support and, at system level, with councils, hospitals and GPs across Doncaster, Mexborough and Rotherham to get schooling, healthcare and housing. It was also heart-breaking – the Home Office could move people on and refuse claims of people I knew to be true. So we got them lawyers and were able to turn round 70% of rejections. It was very difficult. There was no clinical supervision – although I asked for it! – and I burnt out.

Ros Bryar then contacted me and invited me to be part of the first cohort of an MSc in public health she was setting up at City University. So I went back to work four days a week in Hackney in 2003 and did the Master's over two years. It was a vocational Master's with a heavy emphasis on application in practice. My thesis was on post-natal depression – a literature review highlighting how medicalised the approach was. It failed because it challenged the accepted view and I was devastated, but my tutor and another lecturer threatened to resign and when it was remarked I got an A!

Move into health protection

On the programme were two health protection nurse consultants. Again, I knew nothing about their work and had never heard of the Health Protection Agency (HPA), but their work looked really interesting. I went back to Hackney, waited for a vacancy, applied and became a health protection nurse in East London. I settled down, stayed for six years and became a nurse consultant. I could use my epidemiology and we worked in a matrix system, so whoever was 'expert' on a particular disease took the lead on outbreaks. I was the 'expert' for measles. I led on a poster submission one year at the HPA conference and won the prize. It felt like winning an Oscar! I was then awarded the MBE in 2013 for my work before and during the Olympics, making sure there were no outbreaks. It was an amazing experience!

The HPA then became Public Health England (PHE) and changed into a bigger organisation overnight. I thought there might be opportunities for nurse leadership. There had been no chief nurse at the HPA – I had questioned this and failed to get anywhere! There were eight nurse consultants around the country who met regularly – we wrote to the designate Chief Executive Officer of PHE to say there were 200 health protection nurses in the country who needed professional oversight and career development. He approached the chief public health nurse at the Department of Health (DH) and asked her to 'put one foot over' to help. I went to see her about the situation and she said I had talked myself into the job of her deputy. I nearly didn't get it when it was advertised – I went to the wrong venue for the interview, but made it just in time! So I was Deputy Chief Nurse at PHE for seven years with a large portfolio. I co-led on the quality and risk assessment for Ebola and worked on Zika;[v] I was comfortable to be in a skin I never thought would be available to me. I never wanted to be in the upper echelons of management – I liked practical work – but it was the best job and I had a huge amount of independence. I spent the whole time networking and building alliances that still serve me to this day.

Moving to the charitable sector

Then a glass ceiling appeared. Where next? Could I wait for the chief public health nurse job? I wanted different experience. Friends who were in the charity sector said they felt I was ready to come out of government. I would never have considered it but for them. So I became CEO of the Foundation of Nursing Studies in 2019, an organisation supporting nurses to embed innovation in nursing practice and develop person-centred cultures of care. This is the biggest job I have had to do in my life. There is no training for a nursing charity CEO! We have a number of programmes and fellowships and I have been able to double our income and get contracts to support reflective practice and clinical supervision. I am now nearly four years in and working to get the organisation more population focused. This took me to The King's Fund, who were supportive of our work and also keen to get into the nursing sector and workforce. I am now an Associate in Population Health, the first nurse to hold this position. I'm very proud!

An unfinished part of my work is health coaching, which is well developed in America and is psychology-focused.[4] It would be good to have a UK postgraduate nurse coaching qualification which would work particularly well for nurses in the community – supporting individuals in managing their own destiny, their own medication and long-term conditions. This is the future.

My public health journey

When anyone asks what I do, I always say I am a public health nurse. There is a public health lens to all I do. On my public health journey, I have moved from working with individuals to families to populations. I have had a lucky career. If I had not asked questions, met key people …!

My advice to the next generation

Establish your values and keep looking at them. Establish your red line and stick to the red line. Be clear on who you are, your self-worth, what you want the world to be like and your place in it. Think about what your legacy will be. Above all, do what makes you happy. If you want to do something, just go and do it!

Notes

i Lesbian, Gay, Bisexual, Transgender, Queer + others such as non-binary, intersex, asexual people.
ii 'O-levels' or 'Ordinary Levels' and CSEs were the predecessor school examinations prior to the introduction of GCSEs.
iii A fatal human crush during a football match at Hillsborough Stadium in Sheffield, South Yorkshire, England, on 15 April 1989.
iv A Nightingale ward in a hospital is a traditional model, comprising one large room, with no subdivisions for patient occupancy.
v These are both tropical/subtropical virus infections.

References

1. Marmot, M., Allen, J, Boyce, T., Goldblatt, P. and Morrison, J. *Health Equity in England: The Marmot Review 10 Years on*, London, Institute of Health Equity, 2020.
2. METRO GAVS website. Available at: www.greenwich-cvs.org.uk.
3. Metro. Transforming Service, Meeting Needs and Developing Our Organisation. Available at: https://metrocharity.org.uk/.
4. American Holistic Nurses Association. *Nurse Coaching*. Available at: www.ahna.org/American-Holistic-Nurses-Association/Resources/Nurse-Coaching.

Settings for public health practice – useful resources

Acheson, D. *Report of the Committee of Inquiry into the Future Development of the Public Health Function*, Cm 289, London, HMSO, 1988.

Faculty of Public Health, *Good Practice Framework*, 2016. Available at: www.fph.org.uk/media/1305/short-guide_good-public-health-practice_april-2016.pdf.

Marmot, M. *The Health Gap: The Challenge of an Unequal World*, London, Bloomsbury Publishing, 2015.

Marmot, M. *The Status Syndrome: How Social Standing Affects Our Health and Longevity*, London, Bloomsbury Publishing, 2015.

Marmot, M., Allen, J., Boyce. T., Goldblatt, P. and Morrison, J. *Health Equity in England: The Marmot Review 10 Years On*, The Health Foundation, February 2020. Available at: www.health.org.uk/publications/reports/the-marmot-review-10-years-on.

Marmot, M., Allen, J., Goldblatt, P., Herd, E. and Morrison, J. *Build Back Fairer: The COVID-19 Marmot Review*, The Health Foundation, December 2020. Available at: www.instituteofhealthequity.org/resources-reports/build-back-fairer-the-covid-19-marmot-review/build-back-fairer-the-covid-19-marmot-review-executive-summary.pdf.

Marshall, T. *Prisoners of Geography*, London, Elliott & Thompson, 2015.

DOI: 10.4324/9781003433699-16

Part 4

Getting into public health

Fiona Sim and Jenny Wright

Introduction

Having read about public health functions and some of the settings public health specialists and practitioners work within, this section now describes the training and development you might access if you are to embark on a public health career. Whatever your initial background, prospective practitioners and specialists typically train to a common knowledge base and set of competencies. Once trained, you can then expect to make the effort to maintain your knowledge and skills to remain competent throughout your career: that's life-long learning.

There are many different ways to enter the workforce and gain practical experience. By this point in the book, you will have read the career stories of several people who did not follow a standard route through training. This section outlines the more standard or formal routes and what is needed to maintain high standards of practice:

- undergraduate and postgraduate education;
- the UK higher specialist public health training scheme; and
- personal and professional development for practitioners and specialists.

DOI: 10.4324/9781003433699-17

12 Undergraduate and postgraduate education

Susie Sykes; Jennifer Gosling; Dalya Marks; Fiona Sim; Jenny Wright

Introduction

This section looks at what it is like to undertake formal public health courses at a university at either undergraduate or postgraduate level. It offers practical advice on what to expect and what to look for when you apply.

Degree-level courses

Susie Sykes, Professor of Public Health and Health Promotion, London South Bank University

Introduction

This section will introduce options available to study public health at undergraduate level, including degrees, foundation degrees and apprenticeships. It will explore the content you might expect to find within undergraduate courses, information on what to expect, how to prepare and what studying public health at undergraduate degree level might offer you.

Public health undergraduate courses

The number of universities in the UK offering undergraduate BSc degrees in public health has grown rapidly over the last few years, with more than 20 universities currently offering courses. This growth in opportunities for undergraduate public health education reflects similar changes occurring internationally over the last decade,[1] and highlights attempts to develop clearer pathways into a career in public health. Such courses may be titled public health or may be offered alongside other related concepts, such as public health and wellbeing, public health and social care, public health and community studies or public health and health promotion. Other related degrees are also available, which will include content that overlaps with public health principles and practice, including health and wellbeing, health and social care, and population and health science.

DOI: 10.4324/9781003433699-18

Content

Undergraduate degrees in public health will typically introduce students to key concepts and principles, important in the protection and promotion of health and the reduction of health inequalities among individuals and communities on a local, national and international level. They provide the opportunity to explore the links between theory and practice and enable an understanding of the factors that contribute to the health and wellbeing of individuals, communities and populations. Modules within a BSc course are typically worth either 15 or 30 credits, meaning you may have the opportunity to study between 13 and 22 different modules. This will expose you to a wide range of important areas of public health, such as health policy, health promotion, health protection, health economics, epidemiology, qualitative and quantitative research skills, communication, community development, ethics, leadership, global health and evidence-based public health. Modules may also be related to particular public health topics, such as nutrition or sexual health, or to particular population groups, such as young people or older people. Many courses will also offer at least one module focusing on your personal or professional development for employment. Courses are predominantly made up of compulsory modules, but there are courses that offer one or two option modules. These allow you to focus on a specialist area of interest, such as sexual health or substance use, or a particular population group, such as older people. This may be important to you if you are interested in progressing your career within a particular area of public health.

You should expect the course to be delivered by tutors and lecturers who have expertise across a range of areas of public health practice, such as health policy, epidemiology and health promotion. Courses often also invite outside specialists and experts to support teaching, including those involved in the delivery of public health through local authorities. This can provide an important opportunity to gain an understanding of the challenges and opportunities that exist in the delivery of public health interventions and policy, as well as an opportunity to learn about the potential career pathways that might be open to you.

Some courses will provide an opportunity to take on a work placement. This may be a required module, offered as an option for a sandwich course with a year out in practice, or it may be an opportunity that you are encouraged to take up during the holidays, but which is not assessed. These are sometimes organised through the university's employer partners or you may be expected to organise this yourself. Placements may be in a public health team within a local authority or may be within a social entity (cooperatives, volunteering organisations, non-profit institutions) or a non-governmental organisation (NGO). It is a valuable opportunity to develop your professional skills and apply your knowledge, gain an understanding of the working environment and to start to build your networks within the profession. Finding opportunities to gain work experience independently can be challenging, so a university that can provide support with this is an advantage.

You should expect work to be assessed through a range of activities that might include coursework, exams, project work, presentations, practical reports, portfolios and placement reflections. Many courses include a final 30 credit project, such as a research- or literature-review-based dissertation or an intervention planning project. The ability to write reports, deliver clear and convincing presentations, deliver information to a range of audiences and undertake and understand research are all important skills that will be used within public health practice at all levels, so these assessment techniques will all be relevant.

Delivery modes

Most courses are delivered on a full-time basis over three years and are delivered face to face. There are some courses that offer part-time study opportunities where the degree can take up to six years, and a few that are offered as Distance Learning courses. In response to the issues that have arisen following the COVID-19 pandemic, universities are increasingly offering online delivery options or 'Dual Delivery', which may include enhanced virtual learning within the course. Increasingly, courses are looking to deliver content in more innovative and interactive ways – for example, through the 'flipped' classroom, where content is provided to students to study in advance of scheduled sessions, allowing the classroom to become a space for problem-solving and interactive exercises, or through blended learning, which combines face-to face and online learning activities.

Entry criteria

Entry requirements typically range between 80 and 128 UCAS tariff points, including 4/C in English and Maths GCSE. Subject requirements at A-Level or equivalent are not usually stated. However, most courses emphasise that places are offered on a case-by-case basis and students may be admitted on the basis of prior experiential learning. This is part of a commitment to ensure applicants from all backgrounds will be considered, but also recognises that people enter into public health study at different stages of their career and through different routes. Some courses offer an extended BSc (Hons) with a foundation year. This additional foundation year provides an entry route for those who do not meet the standard entry requirements or who are returning to education after a long time. The foundation year provides you with an opportunity to gain the essential skills that are important in studying at degree level and, also, can give you a head start on the subject-specific knowledge. Foundation years are also often transferable to other eligible courses, so they can provide a good opportunity to reflect on whether public health is the right course for you.

Apprenticeships

An alternate route to a degree-level qualification is through an apprenticeship. A degree apprenticeship is a job combined with a university degree. For the majority of your time, you will be working for an employer and you will be studying at university or college for the rest. The apprenticeship is typically 36 months' duration, and the training component involves at least 20% off-the-job training, typically as day or block release. The success of an apprenticeship relies on a strong relationship between the employer, the apprentice and the training provider. The apprentice should expect to receive management, supervision and mentorship from the employer to support their work-based learning, as well as mentoring and support from the university or other training provider.

The Public Health Practitioner level 6 apprenticeship is the integrated degree programme that was approved in England by the Institute for Apprenticeships and Technical Education (IfATE) in 2019. No public health apprenticeships are currently offered in Wales, Scotland or Northern Ireland. There are other apprenticeships that may support a career within public health, such as the level 6 Environmental Health Practitioner, the level 7 Health and Care Intelligence Specialist or the level 7 Systems Thinking Practitioner in England, or the Community Development Modern Apprenticeship SCQF level 5 or 6 in Scotland.

The Public Health Practitioner apprenticeship has been mapped on to the Public Health Skills and Knowledge Framework (PHSKF)[2] and onto the standards required for UK Public Health Register (UKPHR) practitioner registration.[3] This means that once the apprenticeship is completed, you will be included in the voluntary register held by UKPHR as a public health practitioner.

The apprentice must achieve 330 credits of the degree programme and submits a portfolio of evidence. The apprenticeship culminates in an end-point assessment (EPA) which will be delivered by the provider university. The apprentice cannot complete the degree without passing the EPA. The EPA is divided into two assessment methods, which are designed to assess each of the required knowledge, skills and behaviour standards: a presentation of practice with a question and answer session and a scenario-based situational judgement test involving five 25-minute activities.

In 2022, there are just four universities supporting the Public Health Practitioner apprenticeship.[4] You can only apply for a degree apprenticeship through your employer. There is funding available to sponsor the employee's professional development on degree apprenticeships and the university will work with the employer directly to manage this process.

Completing a degree through an apprenticeship can present some very real challenges. The pressures of combining employment with level 6 study require high levels of organisation, efficiency and motivation. However, the benefits of combining study with employment mean that you have continual opportunities to apply your learning within the field and conversely to take your real-world work experience into the learning environment. The opportunity to earn while you are learning and to have your fees covered is another advantage. This scheme is still in its very early days and is likely to grow over the next few years. Information on the universities supporting the Public Health Practitioner apprenticeship training courses can be found at: https://findapprenticeshiptraining.apprenticeships.education.gov.uk/courses/507.

To apply for an apprenticeship, you should create an account on the government's 'Find an apprenticeship' service (www.gov.uk/apply-apprenticeship). You will find adverts for available apprenticeships on this site or you might find them advertised directly on employers' websites. If you are already in relevant employment, you could consider discussing with your employer the option of them supporting you through an apprenticeship. They can find out more information about this at: www.apprenticeships.gov.uk/employers.

Benefits of undergraduate training

For the majority of students, the primary motivation for studying a degree in Public Health is to enable entry into, or progression within, the public health workforce. The public health workforce has been described as falling into three categories: public health specialists, public health practitioners and the wider public health workforce. A public health practitioner is typically defined as someone who 'spends a major part or all of their time in public health practice. They are likely to work in multi professional teams and include people who work with groups and communities as well as with individuals.'[5] The wider public health workforce includes any roles that 'provide the opportunity or ability to positively impact health and wellbeing',[6] and may include social workers, teachers, police, housing officers, doctors and nurses. While entry into the public health specialist category is clearly defined through a formal training programme or portfolio route, entry requirements for public health practitioners are less clearly defined. While a Master's in Public Health has often been seen as an entry-level requirement to the public health workforce,[7] in reality, qualifications required for public health practitioner roles vary, and a study carried out in 2019[8] that included a review of 56 practitioner-level job descriptions showed that only one required an MSc (or MPH) in public health, while the most common educational requirement was for a 'relevant degree or professional qualification' (61%). Despite not having a very clear entry point, the multidisciplinary nature of public health and the wide range of roles through which it is delivered means that a degree in public health can provide some preparation for a wide range of job opportunities in local government, the National Health Service, the voluntary sector or the private sector. Such roles are varied and include, for example, health improvement practitioner, community worker, smoking cessation advisor, sexual health advisor, health campaigner, health communications officer and information/health intelligence officer or analyst.

BSc courses are increasingly looking to demonstrate how the course content can be used to support public health practitioners who are seeking registration on the voluntary public health practitioner register held by UKPHR and this may be something else that a degree in public health enables you to pursue. Practitioners seeking registration must demonstrate knowledge, understanding and application of UKPHR's practitioner standards. A mapping tool has been made available to universities, which they can use to demonstrate how different modules can provide evidence of knowledge against the standards. A list of universities who have used this tool can be found on the UKPHR website.[9] Alternatively, courses may be mapped against the UK Public Health Skills and Knowledge Framework (PHSKF). The framework is often used by employers to identify strengths or gaps in the capabilities of their teams or to design job descriptions for recruitment. A course that has been mapped against the framework will enable you to demonstrate clearly the skills, knowledge and competences you have gained through your study.

A degree in public health also provides an important opportunity to start building your professional networks both with your fellow students, but also with the academics and public health professionals you will come into contact with through your course. Some courses offer students membership to the Royal Society for Public Health or encourage membership as students or on graduation, providing a sense of identity with a professional body.

How to get the best out of undergraduate study

Studying at undergraduate level provides an opportunity to explore the wide range of topics and issues that fall under the banner of public health. This is an opportunity not only to acquire skills and knowledge and progress towards the achievement of your award, but it also provides a chance to reflect on the specific areas within public health that you might wish to pursue as you embark on your career. Seeing this period of study as preparation for that career, you should seek to complement your learning with experience in practice wherever possible. Taking up every opportunity for placements, voluntary work or shadowing practitioners in the field will enable you to apply the knowledge you've gained in the classroom and through your reading and will turn abstract ideas into something far more tangible. This can also be achieved through making the most of the opportunity to build up your professional networks, engage in conversation with those working in the field and see yourself as part of a professional body. Social media, particularly Twitter, has an extremely active national and global public health community where information is shared and topics are debated. This provides the student with an opportunity not only to gather real-time information that may not yet appear in the textbooks, but also with an opportunity not experienced by previous generations of students to contribute to the professional discourse. This needs to be done judiciously and with a critical eye, but can provide a wealth of opportunities and a richness of ideas.

How to seek funding

While some universities offer undergraduate scholarships and bursaries for which you may be able to apply, these are typically fairly competitive and you should look at the individual university websites for information. Regarding student loans for fees and living expenses, you should look at the information provided at www.gov.uk/student-finance, which gives details of eligibility and application processes for each UK country.

Postgraduate education

Jennifer Gosling, Assistant Professor in Management, London School of Hygiene and Tropical Medicine and Dalya Marks, Associate Professor of Public Health, London School of Hygiene and Tropical Medicine

Introduction

This section explores the options for studying public health at both postgraduate and doctoral levels, what you can expect from the programmes and how to get the most out of your studies. For specific information about each programme, you will need to look at each university's prospectus. In what follows, we try to give you a broad overview. However, before you begin looking at what different universities offer, you need to be clear about why you want to study public health.

Postgraduate programmes in public health

There are many universities which offer a postgraduate programme in public health, both on campus and by distance learning. There are also an increasing number who are offering 'hybrid' programmes, with a mix of on-campus and online teaching. Most on-campus programmes take place over one year, if studying full-time, and two years part-time. They often include a period of independent study towards the end of the programme for the completion of an extended piece of work known as a dissertation or project. Most distance learning programmes tend to take longer than on-campus programmes and use a modular format, enabling students to study modules across a period of several years, accumulating credits and building towards the final Master's degree.

A Master's degree is made up of 180 credits. Many universities allow students to study initially for a postgraduate certificate of 60 credits, then a postgraduate diploma for a further 60 credits (120 credits in total). The final Master's degree is awarded on completion of the dissertation (180 credits in total).

Postgraduate programmes in public health fall into two broad types – the Master of Science in Public Health (MSc PH) and the Master of Public Health (MPH). Historically, in the UK, the MPH degree was seen as more vocational, sometimes including a period of attachment to an organisation, and the curriculum would often be based on the syllabus of the UK Faculty of Public Health. It aimed to support students who were taking the first part of their training to later take up leadership roles in public health. The MSc Public Health is seen as more of an academic degree, which focuses on critical thinking, theory, research and evidence. In reality and certainly academically, there is now little difference between the two degrees and MSc programmes will also cover many of the key areas of the Faculty of Public Health syllabus. In many countries outside the UK, there are only MPH programmes.

The origins of public health are as a medical specialty and MSc or MPH programmes will often be found in universities with medical schools. However, the field of public health has broadened considerably, comprising a much more multi-disciplinary approach, and thus many universities that do not have medical schools will offer a Master's in Public Health. It is also now quite common to see public health programmes indicate a specific emphasis, such as Public Health and Health Promotion or Public Health and Nutrition. Other public health programmes will offer students the opportunity to specialise in a particular area of public health during the programme by following a specific 'stream' – for example, Health Economics, Health Policy, Environment and Health or Health Services. The different universities offering a Master's in Public Health will make this structure clear in their prospectus and the programme specifications on their website.

When thinking about which programme to apply for, you need to think carefully about what you are hoping to gain from it – are you studying in order to supplement your skills and develop your career, or are you looking for a career change (whether that be from an existing health-related career or from outside the health sector)? Either way, you need to have a clear idea about what skills and knowledge you want to gain and make sure that the programmes you are applying for will provide them.

The university websites should contain a lot of the information that you need to find the right programme to meet your needs. You should read these carefully before you apply to support your decision making:

- What are the modules on offer?
- Which modules are compulsory and which are optional?
- Are you hoping to study on campus or take a distance learning option?
- Are you planning to study full-time or part-time?
- How much time are you expected to devote to your studies each week, and how are your study contact days scheduled? This is a particularly important consideration if you are planning to study part-time and continue

working part-time. You must make sure that you have enough time to devote to your studies. You also need to check with your employer that they will allow you to reduce your hours in order to study.

• Will you have to undertake a placement as part of your dissertation and what are the arrangements for this?

Most university websites will also have contact information, so that you can ask specific questions of the programme team, if they are not answered by the programme web pages.

Applying for a postgraduate public health programme

Most university prospectuses and web pages will provide clear information about how to apply and what their entry criteria are. It is important to pay close attention to these.

Specific entry criteria will vary between universities, but most institutions will require a UK 2:1 Honours degree, or international equivalent, as a minimum entry requirement. You do not need to have a medical degree or medical background in order to study public health at a postgraduate level in the UK, but do check the application details for specific programmes and what they are expecting – for example, whether there is a minimum period of work experience required. Experience is not always necessary for the application (the programme web pages will indicate any experience that is required, and whether this is a desirable or essential criterion). However, even if you do not have paid work experience in a related field, presenting any voluntary experience will give the admissions team a good idea of your commitment to, and understanding of, the field of public health.

As part of your application, you will almost certainly be asked to provide a statement of why you are applying for the programme. This is your opportunity to make your case for a place. Explain why you want to study public health and what it will provide you in terms of improved skills or enhanced job opportunities. Highlight aspects of the programme that interest you, to show you have done your research in making sure that it is the right course for you. Pick out elements of your previous education and experience to demonstrate their relevance to the programme and your future career plans, but try to avoid just repeating information that is already elsewhere in the application.

Public health is a broad discipline and can encompass a wide diversity of prior education and qualifications. However, if you are coming to a career in public health from, for example, an arts or commerce background, you will need to provide clear arguments for why you are moving to public health to help the admissions team understand your motivation. If you are intending to take the MSc because you are looking for a change of career, it would be worth seeing if you can gain some relevant (voluntary) experience to strengthen your application.

Why undergo formal postgraduate public health education?

As with most professions, a postgraduate qualification in the subject provides a good theoretical and skills-based grounding. It provides the student with an understanding of the essential pillars of public health and the tools necessary to pursue a career in the field of public health. Such tools might include quantitative skills (for example, statistics, epidemiology and health economics), qualitative skills and an introduction to the principles of public-health-focused research, as well as critical appraisal or evaluation and a thorough understanding of the role and importance of the social determinants of health. The education content of the programme will likely provide an appreciation of the wider context in which public health operates, as well as specific skills that would be needed for most public health jobs, be they as an epidemiologist, data analyst, policy implementer, manager or leader of a team, or health promotion specialist. Graduates might go on to work in the UK or abroad for local or national governments, for the health sector, charities or for non-governmental organisations (NGOs), or even transnational organisations such as the World Health Organization (WHO) or the United Nations (UN). The qualification itself will indicate to an employer what skills, tools and understanding of the public health field you have to offer.

As the numbers of students going into higher education increases, the entry level qualifications for many jobs have also increased, meaning that a Master's qualification may be essential for a good entry-level position or to improve your prospects for promotion and career development.

How to get the best out your programme

Having been offered a place to study public health, you need to decide how to approach the programme of study in order to get the most out of it. It is a significant investment of time, energy and money. Without being too rigid, it is a good idea to have a plan for your studies.

Once you have been offered a place, most university programmes will provide some suggested pre-reading. You should try to read as much of this as possible: it will provide a good grounding for when you begin studying. If there is a particular subject that is compulsory and which you are unfamiliar with, or you think you might find difficult – for example, statistics or epidemiology – pay particular attention to the reading provided for these. Most programmes will introduce these at a relatively basic level (unless they have requested prior knowledge at the application stage), but if you are new to these subjects and think you will find them particularly difficult, it might be worth considering finding a free online course, such as those provided by a company like FutureLearn[10] or Coursera,[11] to give you a basic introduction before your studies begin.

Doing the pre-reading can be a useful way of getting yourself back into the routine of studying, particularly if you have been away from formal education for a while: where to do your private study; what time of day is best for you; how you will avoid interruptions, etc. (Get family and friends used to the idea that you need to spend some of your spare time studying, outside the classroom sessions.)

Gaining practical experience while studying

There are advantages to working while studying for a qualification in public health, not the least of which is financial. Postgraduate programmes are a significant financial investment. If you are able to find work or are already working in a job related to public health, it can have a two-way relationship with your studies. You will be able to see direct, real-world application for some of the concepts and skills you are studying; conversely, you will be able to take practical experience into the classroom and use it to test the theories you are being taught and reading about in the literature. Other students without this practical experience are very appreciative of the insights of colleagues who provide practical reflections.

Unfortunately, while it can significantly benefit your studies, there are also pitfalls to working while studying. The transition from 'work brain' to 'study brain' each week can be hard. All programmes will require significant private study and motivating yourself to study after a day at work can be a challenge. Some students also find it difficult not being fully part of the university community or their year group, although programmes are likely to have communication and support groups for part-time students. Seminars and other extra-curricular activities will happen on days when you are not there and there can be a sense of missing out. Finally, while you may be able to reduce your hours, the reality of this over the course of two years of part-time study can be difficult for some employers to manage, with shifts and working hours starting to encroach on study time. It may also be the case that a module you particularly want to study is on a day when you cannot be released from your job.

Funding support

These days, higher education is expensive. If you are not able to self-finance your studies, there are other options. Employers will sometimes provide some or all of the money needed to cover fees, particularly if a case can be made that the programme of study is directly beneficial to their organisation. If they do fund your studies, your employer may expect you to stay in their employment for a period of time after you have completed your Master's degree. UK-government-funded student loans are available for both under- and postgraduate study. These are repayable once a particular income level is reached. For students of public health, there are a number of scholarships available, but competition for these is high. The application pages of university websites will often carry details of, and links to, scholarship opportunities.

What students say they have enjoyed, what you need to look out for,
challenges and rewards

One of the highlights of their postgraduate experience that students comment on is that they have built up long-lasting networks of like-minded peers, many of whom are based around the world. Another common reflection is how enriching the experience has been, particularly in nurturing friendships. Both mature students returning to postgraduate study and those fresh from undergraduate study develop lasting connections that stem from their public health studies.

Students find it particularly helpful to speak to alumni of their programmes or year-two part-time students to signpost them through the degree and offer tips about how to approach their studies, or how to structure their module choices. Many programmes will provide evaluations of modules by former students that can support student decision-making.

Studying intensively for a one-year Master's can be challenging, but also rewarding. Students have commented that they have benefited from organising their study schedule and planning for the year ahead. Many mature or part-time students who have applied the structure of a working week to their studies have managed their workload more smoothly than they anticipated at the start of their year.

The professional Doctorate in Public Health (DrPH)

Those who are reasonably well advanced in their careers and already have a Master's qualification in a discipline other than public health may want to consider a professional Doctorate in Public Health as an alternative to a Master's. At the same level as a PhD, the professional doctorate is aimed at people who do not want to move to an academic career, but still want a programme of higher study to develop or enhance their careers. Rather than a single research project, which is the model for the PhD, the professional doctorate combines taught modules with one or more small research projects and can involve an element of reflection on your professional life. It is more structured than the traditional PhD, but still involves a large amount of individual research and a contribution to knowledge.

Professional doctorates in public health are not that common in the UK. The London School of Hygiene and Tropical Medicine has a long-standing professional doctorate and, in recent years, this has been joined by programmes at the universities of Hertfordshire, Bangor and Chester, among others.[i]

Note

i The sections on undergraduate and postgraduate education are considerably revised and expanded from the first edition authored by Jane Wills and Helen Hogan, to allow for recent new developments in further and higher education, such as apprenticeships schemes.

References

1. Bashkin, O. and Tulchinsky, T.H. Establishing undergraduate public health education: Process, challenges, and achievements in a case study in Israel. *Public Health Reviews*, 38(1): 1–11, 2017, DOI:10.1186/s40985-017-0057-4; Resnick, B., Selig, S. and Riegelman, R. An examination of the growing US undergraduate public health movement, *Public Health Reviews*, 38(1): 1–16, 2017, DOI:10.1186/s40985-016-0048-x.
2. GOV.UK. *Guidance: Public Health Skills and Knowledge Framework (PHSKF)*. Available at: www.gov.uk/government/publications/public-health-skills-and-knowledge-framework-phskf.
3. UKPHR. *Registration Standards: Public Health Practitioners, 2018*. Available at: https://ukphr.org/wp-content/uploads/2019/07/UKPHR-Practitioner-Standards-2018-2nd-Ed.pdf.
4. GOV.UK. *Apprenticeship Training Course: Public Health Practitioner – Integrated Degree (Level 6)*. Available at: https://findapprenticeshiptraining.apprenticeships.education.gov.uk/courses/507.
5. The Centre for Workforce Intelligence. *Mapping the Core Public Health Workforce: Final Report, 2014* (October), p. 4. Available at: https://assets.publishing.service.gov.uk/government/uploads/system/uploads/attachment_data/file/507518/CfWI_Mapping_the_core_public_health_workforce.pdf.
6. The Centre for Workforce Intelligence. *Understanding the Wider Public Health Workforce*, 2015, DOI:10.1093/med/9780198713999.003.0010.
7. Gray, S.F. and Evans, D. Developing the public health workforce: Training and recognizing specialists in public health from backgrounds other than medicine: Experience in the UK. *Public Health Reviews*, 39(1): 1–9, 2018, DOI:10.1186/s40985-018-0091-x.
8. Evans, D. and Gray, C. How important is public health practitioner registration to UK public health employers? *Public Health*, 171: 1–5, 2019, DOI:10.1016/j.puhe.2019.03.011.
9. UKPHR. *Mapping of BSc Courses*. Available at: https://ukphr.org/mapping-of-bsc-courses-2/.
10. FutureLearn website. Available at: www.futurelearn.com/.
11. Coursera website. Available at: www.coursera.org/.

13 UK higher specialist training scheme*

Amy Potter; Katie Ferguson;
Fiona Sim; Jenny Wright

Introduction

This section looks at the UK public health training scheme for those who wish to become accredited specialists in public health practice and eligible to apply for consultant-level public heath posts. It covers how to apply, what to expect from the training and its various stages, including examinations, and includes a personal perspective from the authors.

The UK training programme and personal perspectives

Amy Potter, Consultant in Public Health, Foreign, Commonwealth and Development Office and Katie Ferguson, Consultant in Public Health, London Borough of Islington

Introduction

A Specialty Registrar (StR) in Public Health is someone participating in the national training programme to develop Public Health Consultants. In the UK, the body that oversees training and professional standards is the Faculty of Public Health (FPH).

Public health StRs come from a variety of medical and non-medical backgrounds, but, once in training, there is no distinction between the two groups in terms of training curriculum, opportunities and assessment. Training is usually full-time over five years, although previous experience may be taken into account, and covers knowledge and practice in the three key domains of public health practice: health protection, health improvement, and health and social care services. StRs are supported through training by an overall training programme director and by educational supervisors in each placement. Training part-time extends the duration of the programme pro rata.

---

* This chapter is based on the original chapter produced for the first edition of this book, written by Amy Potter. It has been updated and added to by both Amy Potter and Katie Ferguson for this edition.

DOI: 10.4324/9781003433699-19

Applying for a place on the training programme

The training scheme is open to applicants from medical and non-medical backgrounds. For further information, visit the UK Faculty of Public Health website.[1]

Recruitment to the national training programme takes place as part of a single recruitment round annually for suitably qualified individuals (which includes from the armed forces), usually starting in November, with recruits taking up their placements the following August. The number of vacancies varies each year, but is usually between 60 and 90. Doctors are eligible to apply if they are/will be eligible for full registration with, and hold a current licence to practise from, the General Medical Council (GMC) at the intended start date, have achieved a minimum of two years of postgraduate medical experience by the time of appointment (equivalent to that obtained in a UK Foundation Training Programme) and have evidence of achievement of foundation competencies, in the three-and-a-half years preceding the advertised post start date. Candidates from other backgrounds are required to have a first degree (achieving a first or 2:1 or equivalent grade) or higher degree and demonstrate they have at least 48 months' work experience by the application deadline, of which 24 months must be in a public-health-related field, at NHS Agenda for Change Band 6 or above (or equivalent), with a minimum of three months in the three-and-a-half years preceding the start date of the advertised training post.

To apply, candidates submit an online application form prior to the deadline for the annual national recruitment round and those deemed eligible are invited to an 'assessment centre', which involves written numerical and critical reasoning tests, as well as a scenario-based 'situational judgement' test. Candidates meeting the required thresholds are then ranked and the highest scoring are invited to a 'selection centre', which involves an interview and other assessments of public health skills. Candidates must meet a minimum score from the selection centre and then scores from both centres are combined to produce a final ranked score, used to select candidates for training places.

The training

During the first of two phases of training, StRs typically complete an academic course such as a Master's of Public Health, unless they have completed an acceptable course already, covering core topics such as epidemiology and statistics, disease causation and prevention, social policy, health economics, and organisation and management of healthcare. Phase one usually lasts between two and three years, and also includes some time working in a local public health department[i] and for a local health protection unit providing the public health response to infectious diseases and environmental hazards.

The end of phase one is marked by starting health protection out-of-hours on call work and successful completion of two exams: the FPH Diplomate (DFPH) exam, testing public health knowledge, which is followed six to nine months later by the final Membership (MFPH) exam, where the focus is more on demonstrating knowledge in practice. After passing both exams, StRs officially become 'Members' of the FPH. Meanwhile, underpinning all this is a range of competencies which have to be met throughout training in order to demonstrate a good grasp and experience of different aspects of public health practice, including surveillance and assessment of population heath, the ability to collect and use intelligence, assess evidence and work collaboratively to develop appropriate public health policies and strategies, as well as developing an ability to understand and use different leadership styles to achieve change. All competencies have to be signed off before the end of training and the award of CCT (Certificate of Completion of Training).[ii]

In the second phase of training, and depending on which competencies are still to be acquired by the individual, StRs have access to a broader range of training opportunities. These include placements in academia, with charity sector organisations, working on public health issues or advocacy, with the NHS – for example, working for a hospital trust, or at national level, with organisations like the National Institute for Health and Care Excellence (NICE) or government departments, such as the Department of Health and Social Care. Global and international health placements with organisations such as Médecins sans Frontières or via government departments, such as the Foreign, Commonwealth and Development Office (FCDO),[iii] may also be available. This phase is designed to consolidate core skills in public health practice and develop specific interests to enhance career opportunities. During this phase, StRs take on increasing levels of responsibility and have the opportunity to 'act up' into a consultant level post before qualifying.

Registration

At the end of training, Public Health Consultants must be registered to practise, either with the General Medical Council (GMC), or with the UK Public Health Register (UKPHR), if from a background other than medicine. Dentists have a separate, but comparable, training programme, leading to specialist registration in dental public health with the General Dental Council (GDC).

My route into specialist training – Amy Potter (CCT 2014)

As with many of my colleagues, I came to public health in a roundabout route, taking a while to realise that it was 'public health' that drew together for me a seemingly disparate range of interests: effective management of health services, tackling inequalities in access to quality healthcare and in health outcomes, and the upstream determinants of health, such as socio-economic status, education, employment, housing and community.

As an undergraduate, I specialised in pathology and, while studying the histology and immunology of infection, I began to think about the balance of genetic and social factors which determine why some people are more at risk of becoming ill than others. This led me to a Master's (MSc) in Control of Infectious Diseases at the London School of Hygiene and Tropical Medicine (LSHTM), focusing on low- and middle-income countries (LMICs), which enabled me to explore some of these social aspects of epidemiology, health and healthcare.

I subsequently worked with an organisation called the Tropical Health and Education Trust,[2] which aimed to increase the capacity of health workers in LMICs through training and support provided by long-term links with health institutions in the UK. As a result, I became interested in the role of effective health management and health systems in improving health, and applied to the two-year NHS Graduate Management Training Scheme,[3] wanting to gain practical skills and experience in organisational management and leadership. Through this scheme, and after graduating from it, I worked in primary and secondary care NHS organisations in London while undertaking an MSc in Healthcare Leadership and Management. I had the opportunity to see real changes to services that patients received, including markedly reduced waiting times and shorter post-operative lengths of stay, but after a few years I became frustrated that I spent most of my time 'fire-fighting' rather than strategically improving services, and was also discouraged by the often fractious relationship between clinicians and managers, despite what I felt was our shared vision to improve services for patients. I took a break from the NHS, working with a relief and development agency called Tearfund[4] in post-conflict Liberia, West Africa, managing public health and community development projects.

Returning to the UK with fresh perspective, and wanting to work in a more strategic role, I changed tack from health management to public health and found myself in a remarkably similar job in East London to the one I had been doing in West Africa (only with fewer mosquitoes), working on strategies to support people to improve their health. I managed a local Health Trainer service,[iv] and worked in partnership with primary care, the local authority, voluntary sector and the public in order to increase immunisation uptake, improve care for chronic conditions, address wider determinants of health and reduce inequalities, and discovered that I loved it.

Through colleagues, I heard about the public health training scheme, and the pieces of my career to date suddenly fell into place as I realised that 'public health' gave cohesion to what had seemed diverse topics: strategic action and partnership to tackle the upstream determinants of health and wellbeing outside the health sector, and ensuring that well-organised health and social services are available that meet need, particularly of the most vulnerable in society.

Not coming from a medical background, I had not realised I could apply for specialist public health training until I was working in a public health department with StRs on placement. Although some aspects of being part of a medical specialty were bemusing (What's an ST1?[v] How do I achieve a CCT? What on earth does that collection of medical acronyms mean?), one of the most stimulating things about joining a multi-disciplinary specialty like public health that struck me at the time and throughout my career since is that the variety of backgrounds and interests, and the complementary skills and experiences that we as a body bring together, enable us to tackle the highly complex 'wicked issues'[vi] facing us today, from childhood obesity, to knife crime, to global pandemics, to climate change.

Public Health StRs are a core part of the public health workforce, often carrying out essential projects that other public health staff do not have capacity to do. Specialist public health training offers a fantastic opportunity to work in varied areas and organisations, at increasing levels of seniority, and get the opportunity to try different career options out for size. To illustrate, here is a sample of the work that I was able to do during training:

- I completed a large-scale assessment of health needs for local Community Health Services (CHS), and through disseminating the findings, observed that front-line district nurses and health visitors gained a different perspective on their role in organising health and social care services around the patient, that managers were enabled to use their activity data to check that their services are meeting anticipated local need, and saw my work used as a basis for commissioning services in a different way.
- As part of a national working group to develop new public health guidelines for dealing with typhoid, I reviewed the evidence base for the existing guidelines and made recommendations, which has led to a significant change in the public health management of typhoid cases throughout the UK, ensuring resources are targeted more effectively.[5]
- I worked as a Researcher within the International Centre for Eye Health at a London university. This enabled me to explore a career in academia, to teach on the MSc in Public Health, develop and evaluate training materials and teach international ophthalmology students about health systems on a summer Short Course. This experience highlighted a passion for communicating ideas and supporting others to learn and also gave me confidence about my own public health knowledge and ability.
- On secondment to the UK government department responsible for administering foreign development assistance (then called the Department for International Development, DFID), I provided technical advice on the UK's global immunisations portfolio, helped to organise a high-level global nutrition summit hosted in London by the UK prime minister, and worked with colleagues in Nigeria to develop and appraise options for investment to support polio eradication.

Since completing public health training, I spent four years as a Consultant in Public Health for a London borough, leading a team to commission and deliver substance misuse and healthy lifestyle services, as well as to influence the social determinants of health across the council and local community (for instance, providing public health input to urban planning and alcohol licensing decisions). I was also responsible for the borough's Intelligence function – public health data and analysis – including the statutory Joint Strategic Needs Assessment (JSNA),[vii] looking at local risk and resilience factors and health inequalities. Alongside this, I sat on a Public Health Advisory Committee for NICE, supporting the development of national evidence-based guidelines on topics such as outdoor air quality and community pharmacy.

Since 2018, I have returned to more global health-focused roles, joining the UK Civil Service as a Health Adviser, firstly overseeing DFID's global Early Childhood Development (ECD) research portfolio (for which my previous StR experience of working in academia was highly valuable) and, more recently, based overseas in the FCDO Malawi country office, responsible for our UK Aid-funded health system-strengthening programme with the Government of Malawi and UN partners (the UN Children's Fund – UNICEF, the UN Population Fund and the World Health Organization – WHO), focusing on strengthening the primary health care system, quality of care, and resilience to public health threats such as COVID-19, cyclones and flooding.

At a training event shortly before I CCT'd, I remember discussing with a group of StRs what gave us joy about working in public health, and once we got started, we found it hard to stop. There is an enormous sense of pride in the profession, that we are part of a long chain of historical figures who have made a significant impact on population health, from Edwin Chadwick[viii] to Michael Marmot.[ix, 6] Many talked about the fact that public health as a discipline enabled us to match both personal values and skill set or expertise, giving personal satisfaction as well as intellectual challenge. Effective working in public health is impossible without collaboration: getting things done with and through others, and the diversity in roles, backgrounds, topic areas, actors and organisations involved in public health practice are a real stimulant.

My route into specialist training – Katie Ferguson (CCT 2021)

At school, I knew from early on I wanted to do a history degree, but I had always been a bit of an all-rounder: my A-levels were Geography, Biology and History. Looking back, these seem quite appropriate choices for a career in public health! My first job in the NHS was immediately after A-levels in a gap year before university, where I worked as an administrative assistant in the Planning and Performance Department of the Oxford Radcliffe Hospitals NHS Trust. There was at the time a huge drive to reduce hospital waiting lists (known as the 'Waiting List Initiative'). As well as working as an office coordinator, I supported Board-level waiting list performance reporting and did some basic data analysis for a review of general surgery, which gave me my first taste of NHS quality improvement work. I realised during that year that for my career I wanted a job which was both academic and helped people in some way.

I first got the public health bug while temping during university holidays at the Public Health Resource Unit (PHRU)[7] in Oxford. I was again providing general administrative support and got to proofread reports produced by the team. I distinctly remember reading two reports – one based on qualitative research exploring how best to support South Asian women living in England to manage their diabetes, and another looking at health inequalities among the prison population – and being fascinated, realising the potential that a public health career might offer me.

I studied history right the way through to gaining a PhD in early modern history, but I knew I wanted to explore working in public health more. On finishing my PhD, the team at PHRU invited me back to cover some administrative duties on a short-term basis while I looked for a substantive public health role in London. Knowing I was keen to move into public health, colleagues gave me some project work as part of a JSNA they were working on, and with this experience I landed my first public health job at Westminster Primary Care Trust (PCT).[x] This role was again part administrative, supporting the local Health and Wellbeing Committee and PCT's role in the local council's Joint Health Overview and Scrutiny Committee, and part project support, co-writing health needs assessments. Reflecting on the start of my career, I always advise people not to be afraid to take on administrative roles as there can be opportunities for those with an interest to develop other skills and, through minute-taking for important committees or acting as personal assistant to senior members of staff, you get exposure to a variety of work at senior level which you would not otherwise get until later in your career.

A year into my job, I started a part-time Master's in Public Health at King's College London, while working four days a week. I then succeeded in getting a secondment to a public health analyst role charged with conducting a health needs assessment[xi] on young people with disabilities as they transition to receive adult services. This was a complex project involving multiple stakeholders across different organisations, experience which stood me in good stead for future work.

My next public health role was for NHS North West London as a public health programme manager, supporting a Consultant in Dental Public Health across the breadth of her oral health improvement work with eight PCTs. I moved with this role into local government at the 2012 health service re-organisation, working as a senior public health programme manager for oral health across the three inner London boroughs of Westminster, Hammersmith and Fulham, and Kensington and Chelsea. In this role, much of my time was spent setting up and project managing school- and nursery-based teeth-brushing and fluoride varnish programmes.

Once I had gained the necessary years and level of public health experience, I applied for the public health training scheme and got a place to train in North London. As I already had an MSc, I was on a four-year programme, but actually completed training over seven years, taking time out for children and to do a Darzi Fellowship.[xii] I used the training scheme and my fellowship to complement and build on the experience I already had in public health, which was mostly health-improvement-focused, and to explore a variety of different organisations which form part of the public health system, to give me a greater idea of the system as a whole. For example, I did a local authority placement at Redbridge Council working on the transition of health visiting services from the NHS to local government, infectious disease management at the North East and North Central London Health Protection Team (which was part of Public Health England and is now part of the UK Health Security Agency), an academic healthcare public health placement at the LSHTM, which involved teaching on their MSc in public health, worked on an evaluation of social prescribing[8] and set up a 'making every contact count'[xiii] programme at Tower Hamlets Together, one of the NHS 'vanguards', developing new models of care.[9] My Darzi Fellowship was at Surrey Heartlands NHS Integrated Care System, working on quality improvement for diabetes foot care; and I ended training at the Greater London Authority (GLA), supporting the Mayor of London's health policy work, which gave me a London-wide perspective and where I programme-managed a workforce change programme and worked on the environmental determinants of health, while 'acting up' as a public health consultant. During training, I also spent two years as a regional representative on the FPH's Specialist Registrar Committee, a sub-group of the FPH Education Committee.

Since gaining my CCT, I have been working as a Consultant in Public Health across the NHS and the five boroughs of North Central London as part of the newly established Integrated Care Board, to drive forward their work on population health and to tackle health inequalities.

In public health, I am able to satisfy my desire to be in a job which is grounded in academic practice and rigour, but also have a role which serves the public good, with the ability to have a tangible, positive impact on people's lives and tackle injustices. It also suits my nature as an 'all-rounder' with many interests, as no two consultant portfolios are the same and, indeed, no two days in the office are the same! It is a job with career prospects across a broad range of topics and organisations and there is rarely a moment to get bored, never highlighted more than as a result of the recent COVID-19 pandemic. Furthermore, as I have illustrated through my experience during training, it is also a specialty in which it is possible to train and work part-time, even job share, at Consultant level.

Roles and career opportunities after specialty training

Public Health Consultants look at the 'bigger picture' in tackling poor health and its causes. The breadth of influences on health and wellbeing mean there are roles and opportunities for Public Health Consultants in a multitude of settings, both in the UK and abroad. The following are just a few, but the world really is your oyster when it comes to a meaningful career contributing to improving population health and reducing inequalities:

- working with locally elected councillors and local authorities to analyse the role of employment, housing, social isolation and other wider determinants on the health of the local population, and implementing evidence-based programmes to integrate services;
- supporting the new Integrated Care Boards and Systems to map their population's health needs, recognise their role as an 'anchor' institution for their local community[xiv, 10] and to commission appropriate services;
- working within a hospital, and with external health and social care partners, including the voluntary sector, to integrate health and social care, to improve early diagnosis and appropriate discharge and make sure that services are joined up for those with multiple chronic conditions or social care needs;
- leading the development of evidence-based policy and programmes for national or international charities, government bodies or think-tanks working in national or global health; and
- undertaking research to provide a robust evidence base for public health advocacy, policy and practice nationally or internationally, and teaching the next generation of public health experts.

Skills needed as a specialty registrar in public health

Effective public health practice requires a careful balance between generalism and specialism: understanding the big picture and the upstream causes of poor health and health inequalities, but also having the ability to look in enough detail at the evidence, using analytical skills to figure out the root causes and appraise the evidence for interventions. It requires a love of enquiry and investigation, and of detective work to think about why the situation is as it is, combined with creativity and vision to imagine how it might look in the future.

Much of the epidemiology, statistics and other building blocks that form the foundation of work as a public health specialist can be taught through the MSc, but to really enjoy public health and use your skills to make an impact requires an interest in the 'but why?' and the 'so what?' questions – a desire not only to understand the data, but to go a step further to think about what it *means*, bringing the evidence base to life and making it practical. To lead the change required to improve population health needs an ability to use data to influence decisions, to enjoy communicating ideas with passion and vision and take time to build relationships with a wide variety of stakeholders from community members to local and national government leaders, to work through others and be content not necessarily to get the credit, but to see progress towards longer-term goals, and to seize opportunities to move things forward.

The public health training scheme is an ideal time to learn how different organisations work, experiment with different leadership styles and ways of working as an individual or in teams, practice negotiating and influencing skills and to work with people from a variety of different professional and organisational backgrounds. It requires adaptability and a willingness to get involved; there are always interesting projects, but you may have to be bold and search them out.

How to get started if you are interested in training to be a Public Health Consultant

If you are interested in specialising in public health, there are a number of standard resources available which give you the nuts and bolts of what a career in public health involves, details of the qualifications required and annual recruitment process and an overview of training. The website for each region's School of Public Health provides more details of the training programme within their patch and the FPH website has the contact details of the training programme directors across the UK.

Ideally, before applying for specialty training, to get an idea of how public health is organised in the UK as well as current public health priorities, you can:

- familiarise yourself with key government policies such as White Papers and related policy documents which discuss organisational changes and structures, and who is responsible for delivering which aspects of public health;
- browse the websites of some key public health organisations, such as: the Faculty of Public Health, King's Fund, Royal Society for Public Health and the Health Foundation;
- read journal articles in reputable journals and learn to critically appraise the study design and conclusions;
- follow a vocal #publichealth community on Twitter to see what they are talking about (a great way to keep up with views on the latest policy developments or disease epidemiology, although as with any engagement with social media, a measure of discernment is required!);
- develop a habit of reading the newspaper with a public health hat on, looking for stories about cancer drugs, screening, obesity, climate change, outbreaks of disease, vaccination or funding decisions for health services, taking note of the strength of evidence cited and the experts quoted, often public health specialists; and
- organise to spend time in a local public health department, especially if straight from a hospital-based medical background, and/or volunteer with a local voluntary sector organisation to gain perspective on some of the social and political determinants of health and wellbeing, and challenges to individual and population behaviour change.

Notes

i These are usually in Local Authorities or Health Boards, depending which UK nation the StR is training in.

ii A CCT confirms that a specialty registrar has completed an approved training programme and is eligible for entry onto the General Medical Council's (GMC's) Specialist Register or the UK Public Health Register (UKPHR) – a requirement for NHS consultant practice.

iii Formerly the Department for International Development (DFID), until 2020, when it merged with the Foreign and Commonwealth Office (FCO) to form the FCDO.

iv Local people trained to support their community to get physically active, stop smoking, reduce alcohol consumption and improve healthy eating.

v A specialty registrar in Year 1 of specialist training.

vi Helen L. Walls defines 'wicked' as 'the term used to describe some of the most challenging and complex issues of our time, many of which threaten humans'.

vii A Joint Strategic Needs Assessment (JSNA) looks at the current and future health and care needs of local populations to inform and guide the planning and commissioning (buying) of health, wellbeing and social care services within a local authority area.

viii A social reformer in England in the 1800s, noted for his work to reform the Poor Laws, linking poor living conditions to risk of disease, and improving municipal sanitation.

ix A Professor of Epidemiology and Public Health in London, who has been involved in seminal public health research and policy during his career, including the Whitehall Studies of risk factors for cardiovascular disease in British civil servants, and the more recent Marmot Reviews into health inequalities in England in 2010.

x Primary Care Trusts were large NHS commissioning organisations established from 2000 and dissolved following the 2012 Health and Social Care Act.

xi HNA is a systematic approach to understanding the needs of a population and includes analysis of different kinds of data and consultation.

xii Originally set up in 2009 in response to Lord Ara Darzi's report, *High Quality Care for All: NHS Next Stage Review* (2009), Darzi Fellowships are year-long paid opportunities for clinicians and those in allied health professions to undertake clinical leadership training through an academic course and work experience.

xiii Making Every Contact Count (MECC) is an initiative to train people in undertaking brief health interventions. More information is available at: www.makingeverycontactcount.co.uk/.

xiv Anchor institutions refer largely to public sector organisations whose role and sustainability is linked to the wellbeing of the population groups they serve, and who in turn influence that community's health and wellbeing. Refer, for instance, to the Health Foundation's article, *The NHS as an Anchor Institution*.

References

1. Faculty of Public Health website. Available at: www.fph.org.uk.
2. THET website. Available at: www.thet.org.
3. NHS Graduate Management Training Scheme website. Available at: https://graduates.nhs.uk/
4. Tearfund website. Available at: www.tearfund.org.
5. Guidelines for the public health management of typhoid and paratyphoid in England: practice guidelines from the National Typhoid and Paratyphoid Reference Group 2012 PubMed. Available at: https://pubmed.ncbi.nlm.nih.gov/22634599/

6. Marmot, M., *Fair Society, Healthy Lives*, Institute of Health Equity, 2010. Available at: www.instituteofhealthequity.org/resources-reports/fair-society-healthy-lives-the-marmot-review/fair-society-healthy-lives-full-report-pdf.pdf. And the subsequent Marmot, M., Allen, J., Boyce, T., Goldblatt, P. and Morrison, J. *Health Equity in England: The Marmot Review 10 years On*, London, Institute of Health, 2020. Available at: www.instituteofhealthequity.org/resources-reports/marmot-review-10-years-on/the-marmot-review-10-years-on-full-report.pdf.

7. The Public Health Resource Unit morphed into Solutions for Public Health (SPH) during the health service reorganisation following the passing of the 2012 Health and Care Act. Information available online about SPH is available at: www.sph.nhs.uk/.

8. Ewbank, L. and Buck, D. *What is Social Prescribing?* The King's Fund, updated November 2020. Available at: www.kingsfund.org.uk/publications/social-prescribing.

9. NHS. *New Care Models: Vanguards – Developing a Blueprint for the Future of NHS and Care Services*, September 2016. Available at: www.england.nhs.uk/wp-content/uploads/2015/11/new_care_models.pdf.

10. Health Foundation. *The NHS as an Anchor Institution*. Available at: www.health.org.uk/news-and-comment/charts-and-infographics/the-nhs-as-an-anchor-institution#:~:text=First%20developed%20in%20the%20US,of%20the%20populations%20they%20serve.

14 Personal and professional development, registration, regulation and revalidation in public health

Fiona Sim; Jenny Wright; Jan Yates;
Em Rahman

Jan Yates, Consultant in Public Health – focus on specialists

I have a background in both education and public health and, as such, continuing to learn and develop remains very much close to my heart. Whenever I do an exercise to look at my own personal values and what makes coming to work meaningful for me, 'learning' is always on the list. So, part of this chapter is about a personal journey of learning, what makes us tick and how we keep our motivation, but part is about the professional requirements that public health imposes on its worker bees.

Em Rahman, Head of Public Health Workforce Development
Programmes, School of Public Health, Health Education England,
Wessex – focus on practitioners

The COVID-19 pandemic has highlighted the vital role of public health in the response and management of a global pandemic and the role that practitioners in public health have played. This has increased the interest in public health as a career for many people.

Introduction

Regulation, registration and revalidation are all important in ensuring that public health professionals are appropriately trained, competent and fit to practise.

Some public health professionals are subject to statutory regulation through one of the UK's health professional statutory regulators, such as public health specialists (including consultants and directors of public health) with a medical or dentistry background (General Medical Council, GMC, or General Dental Council, GDC, respectively), public health nurses, school nurses, midwives and health visitors (Nursing & Midwifery Council, NMC).

Many other public health professionals are not covered by statutory regulation. Nevertheless, it is important for the safety of the public that they can demonstrate they have the necessary knowledge and skills to do the

DOI: 10.4324/9781003433699-20

job both now and in the future. Public health pharmacists, as all pharmacists, are registered with the General Pharmaceutical Council (GPhC). Environmental health practitioners are registered with the Chartered Institute of Environmental Health (CIEH) or the Royal Environmental Health Institute of Scotland (REHIS). In public health, registration through the UK Public Health Register (UKPHR) applies to specialists in public health from a background other than medicine and dentistry, and to public health practitioners not subject to regulation from another statutory regulator.

To achieve registration, whether statutory or voluntary, applicants most commonly need to have passed a specified exam or submit for assessment a portfolio evidencing their knowledge, skills and experience. To remain registered, registrants are required also to undertake a self-directed programme of continuing personal development (CPD) throughout their public health careers. Regulators generally levy fees both at initial application for registration and then annually for ongoing registration and maintenance of personal development.

Specialists and practitioners may also participate in professional membership organisations.

This complements, but is not a substitute for, statutory or voluntary regulation. Membership organisations may provide educational or social events, professional recognition through awards for outstanding practice, support for CPD and the opportunity to engage with a wide network of other public health professionals.

The following sections outline in more detail the implications for specialists and practitioners of regulation and personal and professional development.

Professional development

Before specialists or practitioners can become recognised as fully qualified, they need to complete training, which is a formal programme of professional development. It is about learning and developing into a profession that has an established, required set of standards to which its members are expected to adhere. This helps to provide public assurance for safe and effective professional practice.

However, continuing professional development is more than just learning about something or gaining knowledge about a subject or topic. It is about taking the knowledge gained, understanding what this means for individuals and their role and then applying it to the task or job, while ensuring that knowledge and skills are regularly updated so that practice is always up to date with modern expectations and requirements.

Regulation

Public health is a regulated profession and, as such, carries the responsibilities of professionalism. See Table 14.1.

Table 14.1 Rights and responsibilities of a regulated professional

Rights	Responsibilities (obligations)
• To apply for and be appointed to specific jobs in the UK not available to non-registered applicants. • To undertake the activities required within that profession (for example, be granted confidential access to information on individuals in order to oversee a national screening programme population register). • To be supported by the regulator with information, professional standards and systems for maintaining registration. • To explicitly have your level of competence recognised and visible (registration details are publicly available).	• To conform to a defined set of principles and behaviours which include maintaining competence, managing your own health, good communication skills, confidentiality and trust, and honesty. • To accept the sanction of a regulator should you fail to meet these behaviours. • To periodically validate that you remain eligible to stay on a register (five-yearly revalidation).

Regulation of a profession aims to protect the public from harm and does this by setting clear standards and maintaining public confidence in the profession. The regulatory function involves investigation of possible errors, unacceptable conduct and consequent disciplinary actions. Importantly, regulation as a professional confers both rights and responsibilities on regulated individuals, which permits them to carry out their regulated duties.

Regulation of specialists

In the UK, specialist public health is regulated by the GMC, the GDC and the UKPHR, and is overseen by the Professional Standards Authority. To practise at a specialist (consultant) level in the UK, an individual must be on one of these registers. To be entered onto the register, there are two main routes: through a specialty training programme; or via retrospective assessment that an individual's portfolio of public health work, professional qualifications and development are equivalent to that of an individual who has completed a formal specialty training programme in the UK.[i]

Practitioner registration

Registration sits with the UKPHR. Increasingly, job descriptions for public health practitioners indicate that practitioner registration with the UKPHR is essential or desirable. In 2022, while available in all part of the UK, registration for public health practitioners remains voluntary. However, employers are increasingly viewing it as a valuable 'kite mark', hence its inclusion in some role descriptions and advertisements for practitioner roles. You will have seen from earlier sections of this book that the majority of people in public health practitioner roles are not yet required to be registered practitioners.

Public Health Practitioner registration is at the *minimum* level 5 of the health careers framework, which is defined as follows:

> people at level 5 will have a comprehensive, specialised, factual and theoretical knowledge within a field of work and an awareness of the boundaries of that knowledge. They are able to use knowledge to solve problems creatively, make judgements which require analysis and interpretation, and actively contribute to service and self-development. They may have responsibility for supervision of staff or training.[1]

There are currently two routes to Public Health Practitioner registration:

• UKPHR Public Health Practitioner Registration Scheme; and
• Public Health Practitioner (Integrated Degree) Apprenticeship (see Chapter 14 on degree-level courses).

UKPHR Public Health Practitioner Registration Scheme

This route is for those already working in a role that delivers the public health function. The public health function is described as 'improving and protecting the public's health' and working to 'reduce health inequalities between individuals, groups and communities, through coordinated system-wide action'. Individuals will need to meet the following eligibility criteria when applying to a local Practitioner Scheme to complete the programme:

• working in a public-health-related role;
• working autonomously within own area of public health;
• working to continually develop own area of work and support others to understand it;
• contribute to and work collaboratively with different teams and organisations and a variety of professionals;
• have a minimum of two years' work experience in an autonomous public-health-related role; and
• be interested in and keen to pursue a career in public health.

Figure 14.1 provides an overview of the pathway to Practitioner Registration with the UKPHR.

The framework and guidance can be accessed at the UKPHR website: https://ukphr.org/practitioner-registration-via-retrospective-portfolio/.

There are local Public Health Practitioner Registration Schemes available in all parts of the UK. Individuals can find their local schemes by visiting the UKPHR website. Once a practitioner has applied to a local scheme where they will go through local recruitment processes to ensure eligibility criteria

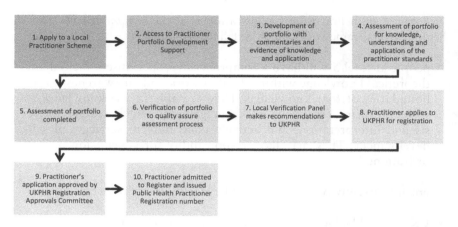

Figure 14.1 Pathway to Practitioner Registration

outlined by UKPHR are adhered to, individuals are accepted onto the local scheme to produce their portfolio of work and evidence against the Practitioner Standards.

Once all standards have been assessed and accepted by their local Assessor, the Practitioner then applies to the UKPHR for independent verification. Following successful verification, practitioners will then apply to UKPHR for registration. This involves the submission of relevant paperwork and the registration fee, which becomes an annual fee paid to UKPHR to maintain registration.

Maintaining registration – continuing professional development

The journey does not stop once registration has been achieved. Regulators have a requirement for registrants to maintain their competence and develop their skills throughout their working lives. This requirement for continuing professional development (CPD) is normally defined so as to ensure all those practising retain competence across the breadth of their current roles, as well as being prepared for their next role should they consider changing jobs. However, we all have our own knowledge, skills and attitudes which influence how we behave in any situation and our CPD must reflect our learning about ourselves, as well as just learning new 'stuff'. All the regulators of public health professionals have their own requirements for CPD activity, which can be found on each regulator's website. But CPD should be seen as a valuable tool for keeping yourself up to date rather than simply as a regulatory requirement.

So what exactly counts as CPD? The UK Faculty of Public Health (FPH), as the standard-setting body for public health, manages a CPD scheme that is a helpful example of how broad CPD can be.[2]

Categories of learning acceptable to the FPH

- learning as part of your job;
- group work, seminars and journal clubs;
- conferences;
- workshops and educational meetings;
- formal courses;
- private study and reading;
- public health audit, appraisal and reflective practice;
- training, teaching, examining and preparation time;
- research;
- organisational development activities; and
- inspection and review activities.

Most plans for developing as a professional are driven by an annual professional appraisal process to review, with an independent appraiser, the whole scope of your public health practice and personal career aspirations. This appraisal is required as part of the regulatory objective of maintaining public safety. The process covers an individual's public health competence and also their fitness to practise in other ways, such as their health and wellbeing and how they might manage the impact of any personal health conditions on their practice. Your own goals and your specific work objectives can then drive a conversation about what development you might need to achieve these and further your career aspirations. You will also consider how you might meet those needs, what support you will require and the likely timescale for achievement. Personal Development Plans (PDPs) often form part of the output of an appraisal.

Now that you have a plan, the development opportunities need firstly to be identified and then resourced if there are financial implications. Many organisations will have ways of supporting their employees' development with study leave time, funding or internal training, but there may be other options to consider as well, such as grants from charitable foundations or awards for which competitive application is required. However, many opportunities for CPD cost only your own time and effort, and not money. For example, NHS England's e-Learning for Healthcare (eLfH) and the Learning Hub (accessible to all health and care professionals upon registration with an email) have many online courses relevant to public health which are freely available to people working in the NHS and social care in England, and there are many more from the UK and across the globe which can be accessed for general public health and for specific topics.

It is also really important to remember that we do not always need a specific course, that we learn through practice and through private reading, watching free webinars from respected sources or videos on YouTube, or team development sessions. Adult learning offers plenty of choice as to how we learn, because people have different preferences and learning styles. So there should be no fixed learning model for CPD.

Perhaps the most important aspects of CPD are ensuring we embrace the learning from every CPD opportunity and that we reflect on our experience to get the most out of it in terms of any difference it could make to our own practice. Becoming a reflective practitioner is an important objective for any professional and that very much includes public health.[3]

Finally, it is worth mentioning that, if public health is your career choice, then seeking out an experienced public health mentor to support in guiding and mentoring your public health development might be very helpful.

Maintaining registration – revalidation for public health professionals

Revalidation is the process by which public health specialists in the UK, along with other health professionals, demonstrate that they are up to date and fit to practise, in order to retain their professional registration. Each regulator has its own revalidation system and, in 2023, some are much more established than others. For example, while UKPHR has introduced revalidation for specialist registrants, it has yet to do so fully for practitioners, where the current arrangement includes five-yearly re-registration to conduct a more rigorous check than at each annual renewal. However, a full UKPHR revalidation process for practitioners is planned.

Note

i See previous section for details of the higher specialty training scheme in public health.

References

1. Skills for Health. *Key Elements of the Career Framework*. Available at: www. skillsforhealth.org.uk/wp-content/uploads/2020/11/Career_framework_key_elements.pdf.
2. Faculty of Public Health. *Professional Development*. Available at: www.fph.org. uk/professional-development/.
3. For more detail, see: Schon, D. *The Reflective Practitioner: How Professionals Think in Action*, New York, Basic Books, 1984; Gibbs, G. *Learning by Doing: A Guide to Teaching and Learning Methods*, Oxford, FEU, 1988.

Getting into public health – useful resources

Organisations

Faculty of Public Health

The Faculty of Public Health is the standard-setter for public health and has information on careers, training and maintaining registration.

Faculty of Public Health. *Careers in Public Health: Being a Public Health Consultant*. Available at: www.fph.org.uk/training-careers/careers-in-public-health/.
Faculty of Public Health. *Continuing Professional Development*. Available at: www.fph.org.uk/professional-development/cpd.
Faculty of Public Health. *Good Public Health Practice*. Available at: www.fph.org.uk/professional-development/good-public-health-practice/.
Faculty of Public Health. *Membership of the Faculty of Public Health Exams*. Available at: www.fph.org.uk/training-careers/the-diplomate-dfph-and-final-membership-examination-mfph/.
Faculty of Public Health. *Policy & Advocacy*. Available at: www.fph.org.uk/policy-advocacy/.
Faculty of Public Health. *Public Health Specialty Training Curriculum 2022*. Available at: www.fph.org.uk/training-careers/specialty-training/curriculum/.
Faculty of Public Health. *Recruitment Information*. Available at: www.fph.org.uk/training-careers/recruitment/recruitment-information/.
Faculty of Public Health. *Reflective Notes*. Available at: www.fph.org.uk/professional-development/cpd/reflective-notes/. (The resources in this section provide practical tips on how to keep reflective notes, including information on how to write reflectively.)
Faculty of Public Health. *Specialise in the Bigger Picture and Help Make the World a Better Place*. Available at: www.fph.org.uk/media/2659/specialise-in-the-bigger-picture-booklet-sept-2019v4.pdf.
Faculty of Public Health. *Training Programmes*. Available at: www.fph.org.uk/training-careers/specialty-training/training-placements/training-programmes/.

General Medical Council (GMC)

GMC. *Good Medical Practice*. Available at: www.gmc-uk.org/ethical-guidance/ethical-guidance-for-doctors/good-medical-practice.

DOI: 10.4324/9781003433699-21

GMC. *The Medical Register.* Available at: www.gmc-uk.org/registration-and-licensing/the-medical-register.

GMC. *Registration and Licensing.* Available at: www.gmc-uk.org/registration-and-licensing.

UK Public Health Register (UKPHR)

This website, as well information on routes to registration at specialist level and maintaining registration, contains information about Public Health Practitioner Registration, including how to apply to a local scheme, how to maintain registration and the benefits to registration.

UKPHR. *How to Apply for Practitioner Registration.* Available at: https://ukphr.org/how-to-apply-for-practitioner-registration/.

UKPHR. *Maintaining Your Registration as a Practitioner.* Available at: https://ukphr.org/maintaining-your-practitioner-registration/.

UKPHR. *Public Health Practitioner.* Available at: https://ukphr.org/practitioner/.

UKPHR. *The Reflective Practitioner.* Available at: www.ukphr.org/wp-content/uploads/2017/11/Writing-reflective-notes-for-practitioner-workshop-conference-pptx.pdf.

UKPHR. *UKPHR Registration.* Available at: https://ukphr.org/registration/.

UKPHR. *UKPHR Registration Standards.* Available at: https://ukphr.org/wp-content/uploads/2019/07/UKPHR-Practitioner-Standards-2018-2nd-Ed.pdf.

UKPHR. *View the Register.* Available at: https://ukphr.org/view-the-register/.

UKPHR website. Available at: https://ukphr.org/.

UKPHR. *Registration via Retrospective Portfolio.* https://ukphr.org/practitioner-registration-via-retrospectiveportfolio/.

Other important bodies

Chartered Institute of Environmental Health website. Available at: www.cieh.org.

General Dental Council (GDC). *Registration.* Available at: www.gdc-uk.org/registration.

GDC. *Search the Registers.* Available at: https://olr.gdc-uk.org/SearchRegister.

General Pharmaceutical Council website. Available at: www.pharmacyregulation.org.

Nursing and Midwifery Council website. Available at: www.nmc.org.uk.

UK Health Security Agency website. Available at: www.gov.uk/government/organisations/uk-health-security-agency.

Royal Society for Public Health (RSPH) is an independent charity to promote and protect human health and wellbeing; an international membership organisation open to anyone interested in public health, including student membership, and provides policy advocacy, qualifications and training. Available at: www.rsph.org.uk.

Royal Society for Public Health CPD: https://www.rsph.org.uk/about-us/cpd-policy/rsph-cpd-activities.html

Association for Nutrition (AfN) is an independent regulator for registered nutritionists. Available at: www.associationfornutrition.org

Health & Care Professions Council (HCPC) is a regulatory body for several health and social care professions in the UK. Available at: www.hpc-uk.org

International Union for Health Promotion and Education (IUHPE) is an independent professional association of individuals and organisations committed to improving population health and wellbeing through education, community action and healthy public policy. Available at: www.iuhpe.org

The Royal Environmental Health Institute of Scotland (REHIS) sets standards, accredits courses and awards qualifications for environmental health practitioners in Scotland. Available at: www.rehis.com

Schemes

Conference of Postgraduate Medical Deans of the United Kingdom. *The Gold Guide: A Reference Guide for Postgraduate Foundation and Specialty Training in the UK*, 8th edn, 2020. Available at: www.copmed.org.uk/publications/gold-guide/gold-guide-8th-edition.

Institute for Apprenticeships & Technical Education. *Public Health Practitioner (Integrated Degree)*. Available at: www.instituteforapprenticeships.org/apprenticeship-standards/public-health-practitioner-integrated-degree-v1-0.

NHS. *Graduate Management Training Scheme*. Available at: https://graduates.nhs.uk/.

General resources

Health Careers website. Available at: www.healthcareers.nhs.uk/explore-roles/public-health-careers. (This website includes lots of information about careers in public health, including real-life stories of those working in different public health roles.)

Health Education England website. Available at: www.e-lfh.org.uk/. (This link provides a directory of e-learning training and education available to public health practitioners, where the vast majority of the training is freely available to anyone.)

Health Education England. *Core Public Health Workforce*. Available at: https://www.hee.nhs.uk/our-work/population-health/core-public-health-worksforce.

Health Education England. *Models of Reflection and Reflective Practice – London*. Available at: https://london.hee.nhs.uk/reflective-writing-models-reflection-and-reflective-practice.

Kolb, D.A. and Fry, R.E. Towards an applied theory of experiential learning. Available at: www.researchgate.net/publication/238759143_Toward_an_Applied_Theory_of_Experiential_Learning.

Public Health England. *Public Health Skills and Knowledge Framework*. Available at: www.gov.uk/government/publications/public-health-skills-and-knowledge-framework-phskf/public-health-skills-and-knowledge-framework-august-2019-update. (This resource describes the key functions in public health and includes tools to assess individuals' knowledge and skills.)

Skills for Health. *Key Elements of the Career Framework v2*. Available at: www.skillsforhealth.org.uk/wp-content/uploads/2020/11/Career_framework_key_elements.pdf.

Yorkshire and Humber Public Health Network. *Resources to Help You Promote a Career in Public Health*. Available at: www.yhphnetwork.co.uk/media/58579/public_health_career_resource_updated.pdf.

Part 5

How to proceed from here

15 How to proceed from here

Fiona Sim and Jenny Wright

Introduction

The book so far has set out a range of perspectives on public health careers. Although the profile of public health has been raised by the COVID-19 pandemic, you will by now have seen that the public health response did not stop with expertise in the technical knowledge and skills of communicable disease control (part of health protection), but depended just as much on so many other core areas of public health delivery, including: research – leading, in turn, to interpretation of a rapidly emerging evidence base, effective health communication, statistical and epidemiological expertise, behaviour modification, understanding of health inequalities, and planning for the huge backlog of healthcare needs for non-COVID-19-related conditions.

This book has shown just a sample of the huge variety of roles on offer in public health, and how to access them, whatever your specific interests and skills. It has also pointed the way to the future and the challenges from new threats to human health, as well as the opportunities and rewards for those working in public health. This discipline – some say it is a movement – will continue to evolve in response to a changing world.

There is no single, straightforward pathway to a career in public health. This is both an advantage and a disadvantage to those setting out on their careers. It is a broad discipline and welcomes those from a wide range of backgrounds and experience, all of which provides the richness of contributions to the public health endeavour. How you start out and then proceed will also depend partly on your own interests and aptitudes; although, as we have seen, there are common approaches and competencies that all public health practitioners and specialists will need.

Attitudes are important

Whatever branch of public health you may plan to work in, a belief in life-long learning is essential. The field of public health and the evidence of what works changes rapidly. The skills and knowledge needed for tasks will evolve, hence the importance of continuing to learn throughout your career.

DOI: 10.4324/9781003433699-23

It is also crucial that you can work with long timescales. Apart from health protection, there are very few times when there is instant gratification in public health practice. Real change in population health status can take time and perseverance, and public health professionals learn to work with interim goals as they work towards their main objective, which could be some years away.

Rewards in public health

Jobs can be tough. There are rewards, however, and not necessarily monetary, although public health professionals are paid relatively well compared with many other disciplines. There is generally little scope for materialism in public health practice. The values held, as you will have noticed from the contributions throughout the book, demonstrate a passion above all for making the world a better place, reducing preventable inequalities, and improving the health and wellbeing of communities, especially of those in greatest need and of those whose voice is not otherwise heard. The reward comes from achievements, often modest, such as getting members of a local inner city community with poor levels of physical activity to adopt healthy physical exercise regimes or introducing an effective vaccine campaign in a low-income country with poor health outcomes and huge unmet needs. Since public health professionals almost always work as part of a multi-professional team, there is the additional satisfaction of working with and learning from one another. These are some adjectives which describe working in public health:

- rewarding;
- challenging;
- problem-solving;
- infinitely varied;
- evidence-based; and
- collaborative.

And contributing to the common good, making a real difference!

Challenges in public health

A key issue to be borne in mind is that, because much of the public health workforce is employed in the public sector, it is subject to periodic organisational change. Governments – particularly following changes in government – seek to improve services or put their particular policy stamp on services. A change of government almost always brings about different policy directions, some of which may or may not aid the public health cause. Change can and should, however, bring about new opportunities and possibilities.

What do you do next?

Now you are ready to get going. The profile of public health has increased enormously as a result of the COVID-19 pandemic, meaning that both interest in public health and job opportunities may increase. Because the public health workforce has been so essential in dealing with the recurrent waves and their consequences, organisations have been reviewing their public health capacity and identifying skills shortages. The pandemic has highlighted continuing public health issues that need to be tackled, as well as new challenges to the population's health.

There are some key steps to begin with:

- explore different roles, functions and settings;
- decide what interests you most;
- think about where you would like your career path to take you; and
- look at whether you need any formal qualifications and where and how you might attain them.

A key issue for those starting out can be lack of experience – even for those with a Master's Degree in Public Health – if they have never worked in a public health setting. If you can, get internships, consider volunteering and, if you have to complete a dissertation for your Master's degree, see if you can include some fieldwork within your research. Some councils offer short, paid fellowships. Another possibility is to find a mentor to help guide you. Those undertaking specialist training are often prepared to help others interested in the discipline. Nearly everyone who works in public health is enthusiastic about their chosen career, so do make contact if you wish to find out more.

When applying for posts:

- consider your CV: how best to present the knowledge and skills, qualifications and experience you bring for each specific role that interests you;
- review your previous experience in either paid or voluntary work, in the UK or overseas, as this could be relevant;
- make sure you understand relevant health and local government organisational structures;
- talk to people: don't be shy to contact people working in the field;
- do your research in advance – think how you can find out more about a job;
- think about factors that make a job more or less attractive for you, such as travel to, and for, work; and
- consider what development opportunities the job might offer you, as well as what you will bring to the job.

Finding your first public health job

You will need to seek out jobs. Advertisements are not all in one place and where they can be found will vary in each UK country. In England, in particular, jobs may be advertised on the NHS Jobs website, Local Government

Jobs website, on individual council websites and in *The Guardian* and *British Medical Journal* (BMJ), or can be found through recruitment agencies. Adverts are now posted separately on the Civil Service website for the UK Health Security Agency (UKHSA) and for the Office for Health Improvement and Disparities (OHID). In the NHS, some Trusts and Integrated Health Systems/Boards recruit to public health positions or seek people with public health knowledge and skills to jobs that are not always identified specifically as public health roles.

It is, mostly, simpler in Wales, Scotland and Northern Ireland, where jobs can be advertised on either the NHS or public health (agency) websites.

Entry level research assistant posts are to be found on university and academic websites throughout the UK.

It is worth emphasising that jobs are not necessarily tagged as public health: that is, public health is not in the title – such as smoking cessation adviser, health information analyst, development worker, etc. Some NHS jobs may be tagged 'population health'. So, it is important to read the actual job specification.

If you are thinking of applying for the specialty training scheme, it would be a good idea first to try to gain experience in more than one public health setting or function. Be prepared that your initial experience could be at quite a junior level, but by learning as much as you can, you will get most value from it, as well as being valued for doing a good job.

Concluding remarks from the editors

We hope by now to have sparked your interest to explore further! Hopefully, some of the stories in earlier chapters have inspired you to think seriously about a career in public health. If you do decide to go ahead, we wish you all the best in your chosen field. And if you have realised that public health is not for you, you might come back one day!

Finally, if you do choose a career in public health at some point in your life, you will never be bored, we can assure you!

Appendix
About the contributors to this book

Fiona Sim. I studied Medicine at University College London (UCL) when public health was a tiny part of the course. Then I trained to be a GP. I soon became aware of my interest in prevention, which was incompatible with my partners' smoking in their consulting rooms! When I spotted an advertisement in the *British Medical Journal* (BMJ) for specialist training in what was then called Community Medicine, which included the opportunity to apply to do a Master's course at the London School of Hygiene and Tropical Medicine, I was seduced. I was appointed to the training programme despite a conspicuous lack of knowledge, but maybe my genuine interest shone through. After training, which I completed when I was 30, I had no game plan and went on to hold a series of senior roles in public health, NHS management, academia and the civil service, including Director of Public Health, Trust Medical Director, Associate Dean of Postgraduate Medicine, coordinator of London's Teaching Public Health Network and Head of Public Health Development for England at the Department of Health, where, among other responsibilities, I led the establishment of voluntary regulation of public health specialists. A strong theme throughout my career, mostly through voluntary positions and research, has been capacity building via teaching, training and professional development. I have been Director of Training for the Faculty of Public Health (FPH), Registrar of the UK Public Health Register and a trainer in both public health and general practice.

One of the great strengths of public health knowledge and skills is their transferability, so a whole world of job opportunities opens for those of us who find the skills and the imagination to use them creatively. Boredom is not an option. Personally, I never really mastered the so-called work/life balance and had many years of guilty motherhood when I tried too hard to get it right and probably missed many of my children's early achievements, but they tolerated their errant parent and never showed any resentment of my career. For 20 years, my main 'hobby' was being joint Editor-in-Chief with Phil Mackie of *Public Health*. I was also a trustee and then chair of the Royal Society for Public Health. Now, when I guess one is supposed to consider slowing down and with the joy of grandparent status, I have a varied part-time portfolio: for NHS England and as a medical appraiser for FPH; I also mentor aspiring medics and teach on a public health Master's course through my visiting appointment at the University of Bedfordshire.

Jenny Wright. When I graduated with a degree in Modern History, I had no clear idea of what I wanted to do beyond an interest in social sciences and trying to make the world a better place. I qualified as a social worker, then moved into social science and health services research and completed a Master's degree in philosophy. This led me to several health and social care service planning posts, latterly at regional health level and in a public health department. I was always focused on how to make services more responsive to population need. When regional health authorities were disbanded in the mid-1990s, the public health department I was in established itself as an in-dependent business unit within the health service, undertaking contract work for a range of organisations, including the Department of Health (DH), local health service organisations, charities and local authorities. It proved a useful training ground in public health and I realised that many of the skills I had already acquired contributed well to the population health work we undertook.

It was during this time I developed a passion for public health development and furthering the interests of the public health workforce in all its guises. I was fortunate enough to take part in the national work involved with the setting up of the UK Public Health Register processes, developing the retrospective portfolio assessment framework used initially in England and Wales. I was then able to qualify as a specialist needing to take the time, along with many others at the time, to update some key competencies and fill in any gaps in my knowledge and experience as I had not had the benefit of being able to go on the higher specialist training scheme.

Despite coming to public health relatively late on in my career, I was able to work with Skills for Health, on behalf of DH, to develop the first UK Public Health Skills and Career (competence) Framework. It was while I was overseeing for DH the England Teaching Public Health Networks programme that I met Fiona. Before I retired, I led the team developing and running the UK Public Health Careers website for the UK Departments of Health, which is now on the NHS careers website. More recently, I have worked with Fiona to produce the first edition of this book and with Fiona and Katie Ferguson to write a history of the multidisciplinary public health movement. I also completed a PhD on women doctors in public health. Like Fiona, as a working mother in the 1980s, I juggled a growing family and a full-time job. The children seemed to survive without harm and my daughter has now become a consultant in public health.

Natalie Adams. Natalie is currently a Public Health Specialty Registrar based in the South East of England and has completed placements working in local authority, health protection and academia. Prior to specialty training, Natalie was an epidemiologist, specialising in gastrointestinal infections and a Senior Public Health Intelligence Specialist in a local authority. She has completed a PhD using data linkage to explore socioeconomic inequalities in risk of and exposure to gastrointestinal infections.

Clare Bambra. Clare is Professor of Public Health, Population Health Sciences Institute, Faculty of Medical Sciences, Newcastle University, UK. Her research focuses on understanding and reducing health inequalities.

John Battersby. John is a consultant in public health working in the Office for Health Improvement and Disparities' Public Health Analysis Unit. He has worked in health intelligence since 2009, when he became the Medical Director of the Eastern Region Public Health Observatory. Before entering public health training, John had trained as a GP and then spent several years running a primary care programme in North Africa.

Joanne Bosanquet. Joanne qualified as a registered nurse in 1992 and very soon realised that public health was her passion. Joanne spent a number of years in this field as a Health Visitor, then in Health Protection. She was fortunate to be part of the London Olympics Health Protection team. In 2013, she became the first Deputy Chief Nurse for Public Health England (PHE) and supported PHE's responses to a number of international outbreaks and incidents. In 2019, Joanne moved into the charity sector as Chief Executive Officer and Lead Nurse for the Foundation of Nursing Studies. She also works with The King's Fund as an Associate in Population Health.

Isobel Braithwaite. Isobel is an ST5 public health registrar, currently out of the public health training programme and based at the University College London (UCL) Institute of Health Informatics while undertaking a National Institute of Health Research-funded PhD Fellowship, focusing on the health impacts of cold and energy-inefficient housing. Before starting her PhD, she held an Academic Clinical Fellowship at UCL and, in her earlier public health placements, worked on a range of issues, including air quality, climate adaptation, equity and environmental health issues. Alongside training, she is involved in work with the Faculty of Public Health's Sustainability Special Interest Group, including linking sustainability and systems approaches with work to address the cost-of-living crisis. Isobel has also been involved in advocacy work related to climate change and health.

Laura Bridle. Laura is a senior midwife working in maternal mental health services in South East London. Laura originally trained as a nurse in public health in Canada before returning to the UK to qualify, and work, as a midwife. Laura has worked as a caseload midwife, in research, and has volunteered with Médecins Sans Frontières. She has an MSc in advanced practice midwifery and a Post Graduate Certificate in perinatal mental health.

David Buck. David works in the policy team at The King's Fund as Senior Fellow in Public Health and Health Inequalities.

Before joining the Fund in 2011, David worked at the Department of Health as deputy director for health inequalities. He managed the Labour government's Public Sector Agreement target on health inequalities and the independent Marmot Review of inequalities in health,[1] as well as helping shape the coalition's policies on health inequalities. While at the DH, he worked as an economic and strategy advisor on many policy areas, including diabetes, long-term conditions, dental health, waiting times, the pharmaceutical industry, childhood obesity, choice and competition. He has also worked at Guy's Hospital, King's College London and the Centre for Health Economics in York, where his focus was on the economics of public health and behaviours and incentives.

Shirley Cramer. Shirley is the former Chief Executive of the Royal Society for Public Health (2013–20), where she was also Vice Chair of the Public Health System Group in England and Chair of People in UK Public Health, a cross-government advisory board on the future of the public health workforce. Prior to this, she was CEO in national education charities in both the UK and the USA.

She is currently Chair of the Rare Dementia Support Group's Advisory Board at University College London and a trustee of Alzheimer's Research UK and Help for Heroes. She is also a Commissioner for the Food, Farming and Countryside Commission.

Tracy Daszkiewicz. Tracy started her career in social care and specialised in HIV. She has over 25 years' experience working in health and social care, across the Civil Service, NHS, Local Government and Voluntary Sector.

Tracy was the Director of Public Health in Wiltshire during the nerve agent poisonings in 2018. This deepened her interest in the role of public health in humanitarian recovery and this is the subject of her PhD research.

She is currently Executive Director of Public Health, Aneurin Bevan University Hospital Board, Gwent in Wales. She is also Vice President of the Faculty of Public Health and a visiting Professor at the University of West of England in Public Health, where she also holds an Honorary Doctorate for contributions to public health. She holds a second Honorary Doctorate from the Open University. She is a Visiting Lecturer in Health Protection at Exeter University and sits on the Board of Trustees for a local Domestic Abuse Charity.

Jennifer Dixon. Jennifer joined the Health Foundation as Chief Executive Officer in 2013. She has been Chief Executive Officer of the Nuffield Trust, Director of Policy at The King's Fund and policy advisor to the CEO of the NHS. Jennifer has held a number of non-executive board positions and is currently with the UKHSA. She originally trained in medicine, and has a Master's degree in public health and a PhD in health services research from the London School of Hygiene and Tropical Medicine.

Durka Dougall. Durka is a senior consultant and programme director in the leadership and organisational development team at The King's Fund, and a medical consultant in public health medicine. Durka leads many population health systems transformation and clinical leadership initiatives across the UK.

Before joining the Fund, Durka worked for the NHS as Head of Population Health and Transformation, supporting 13 health and care organisations to improve the health of 600,000 people across two London boroughs. Previously, she worked for Health Education England as a public health specialist, was a senior fellow in trauma and orthopaedic surgery at King's College Hospital and a senior NHS commissioning manager in London.

Durka holds specialist qualifications in healthcare leadership, public health and clinical medicine, and is a professor of public health and population health part-time across two universities, supporting workforce development and improved practice.

Yvonne Doyle. Yvonne trained in medicine and in public health in Ireland before moving to London to take up a research post. From there, she did numerous jobs in the NHS, Department of Health, academia and the independent sector. She was the Statutory Adviser to the Mayor of London for six years and, as Medical Director and Director of Health Protection at Public Health England (PHE), helped lead the national public health service through the 2020 pandemic. She is currently Medical Director for Public Health for NHS England.

Andrew Evans. Andrew is the Chief Executive Officer of METRO, an equalities and diversity charity based in South East London. He has worked in sexual health for over 20 years, both in the UK and Australia. He completed a Master's degree in Professional Practice and Sexual Health at Greenwich University in 2016 and undertook The King's Fund Population Health course in 2019. Currently, he is also a Population Health Associate for The King's Fund, regularly contributing to the Emerging Clinical Leaders programme from the voluntary sector perspective.

Greg Fell. Greg graduated from Nottingham University with a degree in biochemistry and physiology in 1993. He worked as a social researcher and in various health promotion and public health roles before joining the public health training scheme. Greg worked as a Consultant in Public Health for Bradford, then, in February 2016, joined Sheffield City Council as Director of Public Health. Greg was elected to the role of Vice President to the Association of Directors of Public Health (ADPH) in December 2021.

Kevin Fenton. Professor Fenton is a senior public health expert and infectious disease epidemiologist, who has worked in a variety of executive leadership roles across government and academia, both in the UK and internationally. He is currently President of the UK Faculty of Public Health and Regional Public Health Director for London.

Katie Ferguson. Katie is a Consultant in Public Health working on population health and inequalities across the North Central London Integrated Care Board and the five boroughs of North Central London. Katie started working in public health in 2008 after finishing a history PhD. She has an MSc in public health and completed specialty training in 2021. Throughout her public health career, Katie has worked in a variety of roles in regional and local government, the NHS (both provider and commissioning organisations), civil service and academia.

John Ford. John grew up in Glasgow and is currently Senior Clinical Lecturer in Health Equity at Queen Mary University London and Consultant in Public Health at NHS England. During his academic training, he worked at the universities of Aberdeen, East Anglia and Cambridge. He leads a programme of research focused on what works to address health inequalities. He is also the Editor-in-Chief of *Public Health in Practice*.

Myer Glickman. Myer is a senior health statistician at the UK Office for National Statistics and chair of the Faculty of Public Health's information and intelligence group. His background includes academic epidemiology, research for several medical associations and clinical audit in an NHS teaching hospital. His research interests include small area health variations and socioeconomic inequalities.

Jennifer Gosling. Jennifer is an Assistant Professor in Organisation and Management at the London School of Hygiene and Tropical Medicine. She is an MSc Programme Director and Stream Advisor for the MSc in Public Health. Before joining the School, Jennifer spent 16.5 years as a Practice Manager in general practices across London. She is a Senior Fellow of the Higher Education Academy.

Ashley Gould. Ashley is an NHS Consultant in Public Health and Programme Director of the Behavioural Science Unit at Public Health Wales. He is responsible for the work of the Unit in providing specialist policy, technical and ad hoc support, and developing capability in using behavioural science to improve health and wellbeing. Current activities include optimising policy, services and communications in communicable disease control, maintaining a healthy weight and responding to the climate crisis.

Jenny Griffiths. Jenny is an active member of the Faculty of Public Health's Special Interest Group on Sustainable Development, and a founder and organiser of Alton Climate Action Network in Hampshire, set up in 2019. She has published on climate change and public health.[2]

During her career as a senior NHS manager, Jenny was a champion of multi-disciplinary public health, health promotion and sustainable development. She has been a Non-Executive Director of NICE (the National Institute of Health and Clinical Excellence). She played a very active role in setting up the UK Public Health Register and in developing practitioner registration. She has also chaired several voluntary organisations in Surrey concerned with supporting vulnerable young people.

Shakiba Habibula. Shakiba is a medical doctor from Afghanistan and a UK-trained public health specialist, currently working as a Consultant in Public Health with Oxfordshire County Council. Prior to her specialist training in Oxford, she worked as a medical doctor, a Health Coordinator and a Women's Development Programme Manager for the Afghan Ministry of Health, Oxfam GB and the UN Children's Fund (UNICEF), aiming to promote migrants' health and improve maternal and child health in Afghanistan. She is also an honorary senior clinical lecturer with the University of Oxford. Throughout her career, her most passionate and core interests have been to seek to reduce the inequalities and injustice that afflict the most deprived minorities and those who cannot protect themselves.

Matt Hennessey. Matt is the Chief Intelligence and Analytics Officer for NHS Greater Manchester. His career began in criminal justice as a drugs keyworker and forensic psychologist, but he has since held senior positions in the Home Office, Department of Health, Public Health England and the

NHS. He holds an MBA in Executive Leadership and is an Honorary Senior Research Fellow within the Division of Informatics, Imaging and Data Sciences at the University of Manchester.

David Heymann. David is a medical epidemiologist and Professor of Infectious Disease Epidemiology at the London School of Hygiene and Tropical Medicine. From 2009 to 2017, he was chair of the UK Health Protection Agency and then Public Health England, and during this period he also led the Centre on Global Health Security at Chatham House, London. From 1989 to 2009, he held various leadership positions in infectious diseases at the World Health Organization (WHO), and, in 2003, headed the WHO global response to SARS in his role as Executive Director of Communicable Diseases. In 1976, after spending two years working in India on smallpox eradication, he was a member of the Centers for Disease Control and Prevention (CDC) Atlanta team to investigate the first Ebola outbreak in the Democratic Republic of the Congo and stayed on in sub-Saharan Africa for 13 years in various field research positions on Ebola, monkeypox, Lassa Fever, malaria and other tropical diseases. He has published over 275 peer-reviewed articles and book chapters, is editor of the *Control of Communicable Diseases Manual,* and is an elected member of the UK Academy of Medical Sciences and the US National Academy of Medicine. In 2009, he was named an Honorary Commander of the Most Excellent Order of the British Empire for services to global health.

Manuelle Hurwitz. Manuelle is the Director of Programmes at the International Planned Parenthood Federation (IPPF). Prior to joining IPPF, Manuelle worked as a Research Officer for the University of Oxford. Manuelle has a BA in Social Anthropology and a MSc in Medical Demography. She has a special interest in working towards sexual and reproductive rights, social justice and equity of access in health.

Leena Inamdar. Leena is a public health physician with over 25 years' experience, including working in the UK and India. She is a specialist in communicable disease control and has led incident and outbreak response, including pandemic response, working both at the front-line operational level and the policy and strategic level.

She currently works at the UK Health Security Agency, leading on global health. Her role involves supporting low- and middle-income countries in Africa and Asia to strengthen the control of their infectious disease, including capacity building for early detection of new variants of SARS-CoV-2 and other new and emerging pathogens.

Leena has worked for US Centers for Disease Control and Prevention (CDC) in India on antimicrobial surveillance and on vaccine policy as a Senior Advisor, Evidence to Policy, for the Ministry of Health in India. She has served as a Technical Advisor for the World Health Organization on health system strengthening and capacity-building projects. She is an experienced public health trainer for the UK Public Health Specialist training programme.

Anne Johnson. Dame Anne Johnson is Professor of Infectious Disease Epidemiology at University College London, Co-Director of UCL Health of the Public and President of the UK Academy of Medical Sciences. After training in medicine in Cambridge and Newcastle Universities, she specialised in epidemiology and public health. Her career has focused on research into the epidemiology and prevention of HIV and sexually transmitted infections, as well as other infections such as influenza, Ebola, antimicrobial resistance and COVID-19. She is a former member of the Department for Environment, Food & Rural Affairs Adaptation Sub-Committee of the Committee on Climate Change and a former Governor of the Wellcome Trust. She chairs the UK Committee for Strategic Coordination of Health of the Public Research.

Andrew Jones. Andrew is Deputy National Director for Health Protection and Screening Services in Public Health Wales and is the current chair of UK Public Health Register (UKPHR).

Andrew initially qualified and worked in environmental health. In 2003, he became the first generalist specialist to register with the UKPHR. Andrew has held leadership posts at local and national level in Wales, including as a consultant in public health, Executive Director of Public Health and Director of Health Protection and Microbiology.

Phil Mackie. Phil is a Consultant in Public Health with NHS Grampian. Before this, he was the lead consultant for the Scottish Public Health Network. He has held a range of academic roles and is currently an Honorary Professor in Public Health at the University of Aberdeen. He is a former joint Editor-in-Chief of the journal *Public Health*.

Dalya Marks. Dalya is Associate Professor of Public Health at the London School of Hygiene and Tropical Medicine. She is an academic and public health practitioner with extensive experience of working across London. She is driven by a desire to address the health inequalities in our society and ensure that her research is of relevance to policy makers and planners.

As part of this function, she is co-investigator on a National Institute for Health and Care Research (NIHR) Health Determinant Research Collaboration, part of the NIHR School for Public Health Research and academic lead for patient and public involvement in the NIHR ARC for North Thames. She is also a Programme Director on the MSc in Public Health at the London School of Hygiene and Tropical Medicine.

Martin McKee. Martin is Professor of European Public Health at the London School of Hygiene and Tropical Medicine, where he created the European Centre on Health of Societies in Transition (ECOHOST), a World Health Organization Collaborating Centre, and is also Research Director of the European Observatory on Health Systems and Policies.

Dona Milne. Dona has worked as a Consultant in Public Health since 2010. Prior to joining Lothian as Director of Public Health and Health Policy, Dona was a Director of Public Health in Fife, following a six-year period as Deputy Director in Lothian. She has worked in children and young people's health and education within local authorities, the voluntary sector, Scottish Government and the NHS.

Dona is a Fellow of the Faculty of Public Health and Honorary Fellow of the Faculty of Sexual and Reproductive Health. Her career has taken her to Young Women's Christian Association (YWCA) Scotland as Deputy Director, and for seven years she led the 'Healthy Respect' National Demonstration Project. In 2008, Dona was seconded to Scottish Government and led the H1N1 vaccination campaign following a period in sexual and reproductive health and HIV policy.

Oluwakemi Olufon. Oluwakemi is Principal Health Protection Practitioner with the UK Health Security Agency. She has an established career in public health nursing and received the honorary title of Queen's Nurse for her contribution to public health in 2018. She has held various roles within public health and health protection, and her particular interests are outbreak management and pandemic preparedness. In her current role, she is responsible for undertaking rapid investigations at local, regional and national levels where an outbreak has occurred. Oluwakemi is also a practitioner member of the Faculty of Public Health and is passionate about the prevention of communicable disease in the wider population.

Yeyenta Osasu. Yeyenta is the National Lead for the Community Pharmacy Blood Pressure Check service within the Pharmacy Integration team at NHS England. Her role involves working across systems and sectors to support the reduction of health inequalities at national and system levels through hypertension case finding and blood pressure optimisation programmes. She is a Health Education England national population health fellow and holds a PhD from the Academic Unit of Primary Care, University of Sheffield, where she is also an Honorary Research Fellow. Previous roles include medicines optimisation in clinical pharmacy, and Regional Health Equity Improvement Manager (North East and Yorkshire).

Anita Parkin. Anita worked in various public health roles for 30 years in England, 20 of them as a Director of Public Health in the South East, Yorkshire and London. She is now a part-time Director of Population Health in a large London NHS community trust, a population health associate at The King's Fund and a Local Government Association associate.

Mahendra G. Patel. Mahendra is a nationally and internationally renowned pharmacist with professorial roles in the UK, the USA and, until recently, Malaysia. He has served on the Royal Pharmaceutical Society as national board member and Treasurer, and is an International Teaching and Faculty Board Member for the Bioethics UN Educational, Scientific and Cultural Organization (UNESCO) programme.

Mahendra's work focuses on improving health and health inequalities in ethnic minority and underserved communities. As Pharmacy, Inclusion and Diversity Lead at University of Oxford, he supports the recruitment of these communities into clinical trials.

Mahendra is a national and international award-winner and was made Officer of the British Empire in 2022.

David Pencheon. David Pencheon is a UK-trained doctor and founder Director of the Sustainable Development Unit (SDU) for NHS England and Public Health England, which was established in 2007 and has now grown into the 'Greener NHS'. He is currently an Honorary Professor and an Associate at the Medical and Health School, University of Exeter, an Advisory Group member and associate with the Wellcome Centre for Cultures and Environments of Health, and a collaborator with the European Centre for Environment and Health and the Global Systems Institute, both at the University of Exeter. He is also a Commissioner on the Food, Farming and Countryside Commission.

He has held appointments at University College London (UCL), and is a visiting Professor at the Centre for Environment and Sustainability (CES) at the University of Surrey and an Adjunct Professor at Monash University in Melbourne, 2020. In 2018, he was a visiting scholar at the University of Sydney, Australia.

Previously, he was Director of the Public Health Observatory in Cambridge from 2001 to 2007. He has worked as a clinical doctor in the NHS, a joint Director of Public Health in North Cambridgeshire, a Public Health Training Director with the NHS R&D programme, and in rural China in the early 1990s with Save the Children Fund (UK).

He was awarded the OBE in the 2012 New Year's Honours List for services to public health and to the NHS, and in 2020 was awarded the *British Medical Journal* (BMJ) award for outstanding contribution to health.

Amy Potter. Amy Potter is currently working as a Health Adviser for the UK Foreign, Commonwealth and Development Office. She studied Natural Sciences (Pathology) as an undergraduate and has Master's degrees in Control of Infectious Diseases (2004) and Healthcare Leadership and Management (2008). She qualified as a registered Consultant in Public Health in 2014, having completed the national training programme and the Faculty of Public Health professional examinations.

Sarah Price. Sarah is the Chief Officer for Population Health and Inequalities and Deputy Chief Executive of NHS Greater Manchester Integrated Care with responsibility for population health improvement, screening and immunisation, primary care, adult social care transformation, data and intelligence for the system, including wider transformation.

Before taking up her current role, Sarah was Chief Officer for Greater Manchester's Health and Social Care Partnership through the pandemic and the Executive Lead for Population Health and Commissioning, developing and leading the implementation of a £30 million programme to improve health outcomes in the City Region.

Previous to this, Sarah was the Chief Officer at Haringey Clinical Commissioning Group for four years. Sarah championed the development of new models of care for people in Haringey and changed the way key services are commissioned, focusing on outcomes.

She was the first non-medical Director of Public Health in London in 2003, working for Islington Primary Care Trust and the London Borough of Islington. She was the senior lead on public health across North Central

London, responsible for the delivery of the transition programme for the changes outlined in the 2012 Health and Social Care Act.

Em Rahman. Em leads public health workforce development for Health Education England in South East England. His previous experience includes behaviour change services development, capacity building, sexual health and community development working at local, regional and national levels. Em leads the Wessex UKPHR Public Health Practitioner Scheme. A registered Health Promotion Practitioner with the International Union for Health Promotion and Education, Em is passionate about supporting individuals and workforces, through training and education, in their public health development and helping them recognise the role they have in addressing health inequalities.

Mala Rao. Professor Mala Rao is Director, Ethnicity and Health Unit and Senior Clinical Fellow, Department of Primary Care and Public Health, Imperial College London. Her public health career has spanned practice, policy, research and teaching mainly in the UK, and has taken her from the local to national and global arenas. Her most notable achievements have been in the areas of workforce development for public health, strengthening health systems and planetary health.

David Roberts. David has a background in internal medicine, having worked in hospitals in Birmingham and Cardiff prior to training in public health. While training in public health, David completed placements in health protection and at national specialist centres, with specialist training in Field Epidemiology. He now works as a Consultant in Health Protection with the UK Health Security Agency. He lives with his wife and two sons in Oxfordshire.

Giri Shankar. Giri is the Director for Health Protection at Public Health Wales. He has 24 years' experience in the field of communicable disease/infectious disease control and public health. His special interests are in field epidemiology, outbreak investigation, emergency preparedness, healthcare-associated infections, sexually transmitted infections, risk-communications-led behaviour change and research and evaluation. He has published a number of scientific articles in peer-reviewed journals. He obtained his undergraduate medical degree from Bangalore University, India, followed by an MD in Community Medicine. He then moved to the UK and completed higher specialist training in public health.

During the pandemic, he was one of the Incident Directors for the COVID-19 response. He is an expert member of the Welsh Technical Advisory Cell (TAC) that provides advice to Welsh Ministers on various aspects of pandemic control. In recognition of his services to public health during the COVID-19 pandemic, he was awarded an MBE in 2021.

Cathy Steer. Prior to a career in public health, Cathy worked as a dietitian in various hospital and community roles. She started her career in NHS Ayrshire and Arran before moving to take on senior dietetic roles in Leicestershire Health and North Tyneside Health Authorities. After moving to Highland to take up a dietetic post in mental health services, Cathy joined NHS Highland Public Health team in 1995 as a Heart Health Officer. She took on a Senior Health Improvement role in 1999 and set up and ran a programme of work on tobacco and smoking cessation. She has worked as Head of Health Improvement in NHS Highland since 2007 and provides leadership to and oversight of a broad range of Health Improvement programmes. Cathy's main interests are health inequalities, partnership working for health, community planning, the wider determinants of health and workforce development.

Susie Sykes. Susie is Professor of Public Health and Health Promotion in the Institute of Health and Social Care at London South Bank University. She has a background in public health practice in both the voluntary and public sectors before moving into academic public health 20 years ago. She is the Chief Investigator of PHIRST (Public Health Intervention Responsive Studies Team) South Bank, a National Institute of Health and Care Research-funded, UK-wide innovative inter-disciplinary Evaluation Centre, established to co-produce and evaluate locally led public health interventions. Susie also established and leads PHET@LSBU (public health education and training), which offers a programme of continuing professional development supporting public health practitioners through to registration. Susie's areas of research interest focus on health literacy, community-focused public health, intervention evaluation and workforce development, and she is involved in a number of collaborative research projects in the UK and internationally. She has written and presented extensively on health literacy with a particular interest in critical health literacy.

Christopher Whitty. Chris is Chief Medical Officer for England. He worked previously as Chief Scientific Advisor to the Department of Health and Social Care and was Head of the National Institute for Health and Care Research, as well as Professor of Public and International Health at the London School of Hygiene and Tropical Medicine.

A clinical epidemiologist, he has worked clinically and in public health and clinical research in the UK, Asia and Africa, and is still a practising NHS physician.

Jan Yates. Jan Yates has a background in teaching and moved into public health, completing specialist training in 2008. She worked for three years as a Director of Public Health. Following that, she has held national and regional leadership positions in public health education and assuring the quality of public health screening programmes at regional and national levels. Jan is also a Director in a company providing leadership development courses.

References

1. *Fair Society, Healthy Lives*, The Marmot Review, Institute of Health Equity, 2010.
2. Faculty of Public Health. *Sustaining a Healthy Future: Taking Action on Climate Change*, 2008; Griffiths, J. (lead editor), Adshead, F., Rao, M. and Thorpe A. *The Health Practitioner's Guide to Climate Change: Diagnosis and Cure*, London, Earthscan, 2009.

Index

Page numbers in italics represent figures. Page numbers followed by 'n' represent notes.